30 Needles Constellation Acupuncture

30 Needles Constellation Acupuncture

Dr Jerzy George Dyczynski

dyczymskitelehealth.co

CONTENTS

You should always seek advice from a qualified healthcare professional

Information in this book is intended as general summary information that is made available to the public. It is not intended to provide specific medical advice, or to take the place of a qualified healthcare professional. Information resources are designed to help readers to better understand their own health and diagnosed conditions. You are urged to consult with qualified health care providers for diagnosis and treatment and for answers to personal health care questions.

This book is dedicated to all who love medicine and its contemporary, traditional, and ancient knowledge. Medicine is both an art and a spiritual practice.

This book is a guide for those who are on a journey toward perfect health, seeking the harmonious balance of heart, mind, soul, and body. It is for those who understand that true well-being is a matter of holistic medicine.

I thank you all, thousands upon thousands of my friends and patients, for your trust in acupuncture, traditional medicine, combined with my expertise in cardiology and my profound medical knowledge.

Thank you Amelia, Bella, Sarah, Joley, Laura, Kerstin, Dirk and Klaus for the pictures illustrating this book.

I acknowledge our Chinese teachers, scientists, and friends, and I am filled with gratitude for the precious traditional medicine knowledge and ancient wisdom of acupuncture that they have shared with my wife, Angela, and me.

It is also dedicated to my wife, Angela, a health professional, psychologist, and specialist in modern psychosomatics, trained in Germany, the US, and Beijing, who is genuinely the co-author with many excellent insights in acupuncture and traditional medicine. Thank you, Angela, from my heart.

The origin of the 30 Needles Acupuncture

Jesus said to them, "Surely you will quote this proverb to me: 'Physician, heal yourself!' Luke Chapter 4, Verse 23.

The origin of the 30 Needles Constellation Acupuncture.

My introduction to acupuncture began with my beautiful and divine wife, Angela. It was Angela who first introduced me to complementary medicine, particularly acupuncture. Being curious about what acupuncture is, I have accompanied Angela to a renowned acupuncturist in West Germany, who was not only highly sought after in acupuncture but also a distinguished professor, lecturing on acupuncture and traditional medicine at the Medical University of Frankfurt in West Germany.

For the first time, I personally experienced the remarkable effects of acupuncture needles. I was amazed and astonished by the significant and profound impact of acupuncture on my body. After an acupuncture treatment, I felt renewed in my body, mind, and soul. I also notice that the needles activated my body's self-organizing system. My minor skin cuts healed much quicker, and my dentist told me that my gums looked at their best, with no signs of inflammation.

Feeling both moved and grateful, I began my journey from an internal medicine specialist to a holistic cardiologist, fully trained in acupuncture, a transformation that spanned over 30 years, for which I remain deeply thankful.

I used to travel all over the world with a bag full of medicines. I had pills for cough, for infection, antibiotics, and all possible symptoms I could experience during my journeys.

Three months after our first intense encounter, we were married in Oberstdorf, Allgäu—a picturesque mountain town with impressive alpine nature that left a profound impression on me. It was *love at first sight.* Our honeymoon destination was Greece. Anticipating potential health concerns, I prepared extensively by packing medications for cough, infection, antibiotics, and other possible ailments. However, upon noticing my black bag, Angela disposed all of it and, with a smile, gave me a bottle of Swedish Bitters as a comprehensive all-around remedy.

After we returned home from our honeymoon, I felt convinced to practice the traditional medicine from day one. We started making acupuncture on each other in a way we thought was good. We purchased a textbook on acupuncture and needles, and then practiced acupuncture on each other with the best intentions. It did not take long for our enthusiasm to face a humbling reality—we both fell ill not long after.

We intuitively understood that acupuncture is a complex field that requires extensive knowledge and expertise.

We have been reading books by Paramahansa Yogananda with great joy as part of our daily spiritual training. His profound wisdom, encapsulated in a quote we stumbled upon, resonated deeply with us: *"As long as the power in the eye enables you to behold the stars, as long as you enjoy God's sunshine and breathe His air, so long you will yearn for knowledge".*

We decided to go to China to learn about the origin of acupuncture, the art of inserting the needles in the right points and in the correct constellation."

We booked a special program at the International Acupuncture Training Center for thousands of US dollars. We took our 2-year-old daughter, Fatima, with us. We had booked a suite at the Kempinski Hotel, which was under construction at the time, for $70 a day and boarded the Air China aircraft en route to Beijing.

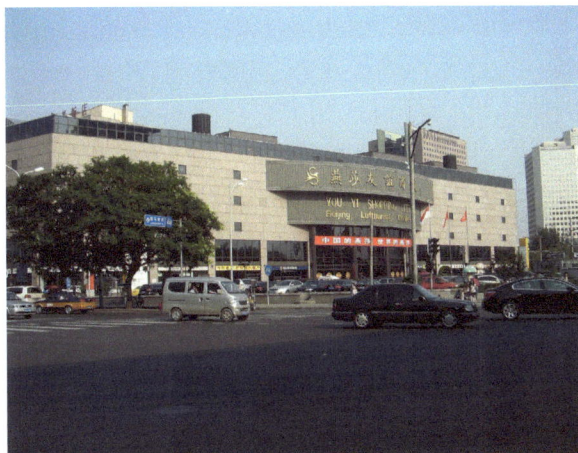

Picture 1. The Kempinski Hotel Beijing.
By WhisperToMe - Own work, CC0,
https://commons.wikimedia.org/w/index.php?curid=22221560

Our arrival in Beijing was a notable and spectacular experience. The early 1990s presented a genuine and striking image of China, characterized by the presence of dust and smog that defined the city's initial gray impression. During our transfer from the airport, we observed a truck transporting half of a swine in the open; as the vehicle accelerated, one of its wheels detached, prompting the driver to pull off the road efficiently.

We arrived at the hotel, and our translator and interpreter were waiting for us along with about ten other people. We did not know that the Chinese people enjoy spending time together, visiting, and working together. It became evident that group activities and collective engagement are valued aspects of Chinese culture.

Our hotel was spacious, modern, and rewarding. We need to accommodate about 20 people in our suite for the first meeting with our Chinese friends. They took our Fatima in their arms, not believing that she had blonde hair, and passed her from one to another, shouting and cherishing Fatima with great joy. It was a reception from the heart...

The Department of Acupuncture at the University of Traditional Medicine in Beijing was about a 40-minute taxi ride from our hotel, and we spent all our mornings there learning the theory and the framework of traditional medicine. Every day we returned to our hotel to meet our daughter and her second "mum", Miss Fong, and we had lunch together. In the afternoon, we traveled to the Xuanwu Hospital for Acupuncture and Traditional Chinese Medicine to practice acupuncture with the renowned Dr. Li.

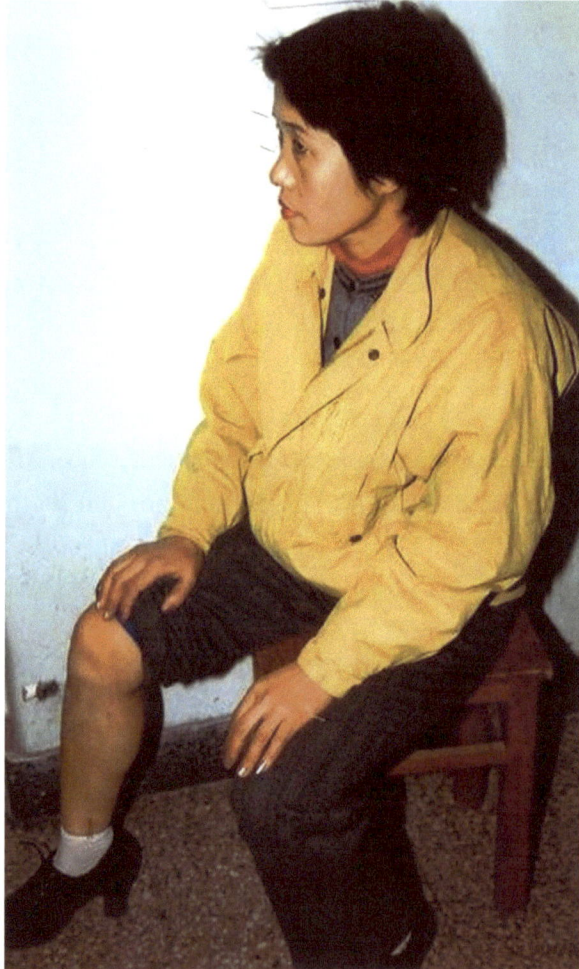

**Picture 2. It shows the acupuncture treatment at the
Xuan-Wu Hospital in Beijing.**

Four Famous Acupuncture Schools in China.

There were four renowned acupuncture schools in China, each with a rich history predating the creation of the Universities for Traditional Medicine in the 1960s. These schools, located in Beijing, Chengdu, Shanghai, and Guangdong, are pillars of the traditional Chinese acupuncture treatment.

Each of these institutions developed distinct methods and unique treatment approaches in acupuncture, many of which are not documented in standard textbooks. The fundamental needle techniques used in these schools were traditionally passed down verbally, a privilege reserved for trusted students.

I received personal training from Dr Li in 1991, 1992, and 1997 at the Xuan-Wu Hospital, the teaching hospital of the University of Traditional Chinese Medicine in Beijing. This personal connection with Dr. Li, a distinguished member of the Beijing School of Acupuncture, one of the most prominent schools in China, was instrumental in my introduction to this special technique of using a 30-Needle Constellation Acupuncture for stress reduction.

Since I completed Dr Li's acupuncture training, I have observed in my medical practice that this particular constellation is not only unique but also highly effective. It has been highly beneficial in a variety of medical conditions I encountered as a medical doctor, giving me a sense of reassurance and confidence in applying acupuncture treatments.

Inspired by my wife, Angela, and our Qi-gong teacher, Prof. Liu, from the Department of Qi-gong at the University of Traditional Chinese Medicine in Beijing, I added an introduction to abdominal breathing to the 30 Needles Constellation Acupuncture treatment.

2

Intro to Acupuncture

The part can never be well unless the whole is well. Plato.

Acupuncture is a safe and holistic treatment. It includes inserting ultra-fine, sterile needles into the skin at precisely defined acupuncture points. In the meaning of bio-energetics, these are the open entry points into your body. The 14 energy channels accessible for acupuncture have 361 classical entry points. There are 40 extra-points located differently from the 361 points at the 14 energy channels, and there is a great number of so-called Ashi points. The Ashi acupuncture points, also known as 'Ah, yes!' points, are non-fixed, sensitive areas on the body that are discovered through palpation and visual inspection, rather than by learning their anatomical location. These points play an essential role in acupuncture practice, as they are the areas where you feel pain or over-sensitivity when touched. They develop because your internal organs repeatedly send messages via spinal nerves to your skin and muscles, informing you through the body's surface about any internal dysfunction. This special communication between the inferior part of your body and external structures, such as skin, connective tissue, and muscles, was first described by Dr. Henry Head, a Neurologist from London in the 1890s, and named after him as the Head's zones.

Ashi points, unlike the classical entry points, do not have a defined anatomical location. They are the tender points where you feel tenderness or over-sensitivity when touched. The term 'Ashi' is a traditional combination of 'Au,' which represents your possible exclamation in response to touching when the point is found, and 'shi,' which is the Chinese person's agreement and confirmation to a question asked by the acupuncturist Is this the tender spot?

Acupuncture not only clears your energy channels and restores internal organ functionality but also increases your body awareness by stimulating the "small man" or "small woman" blueprint contained in your brain. This heightened awareness helps you better understand your body's needs. It also activates its self-organizing system; for example, it boosts the release of your stem cells and accelerates detox, to maintain your perfect health.

The immediate, holistic experience of the great benefits of the 30 Needles Constellation Acupuncture is a life-changing experience. It takes you instantly from the turmoil of your mind to the present moment and to the awareness of your body. Acupuncture with this specific 30 Needles Constellation is a unique, integral, holistic and rapid path to healing and to your well-feeling.

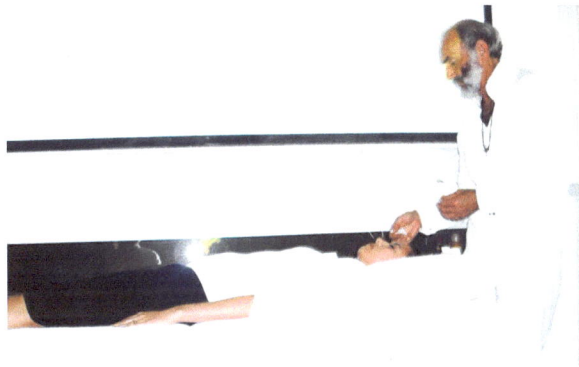

Picture 3. It displays an acupuncture treatment in clinical setting.

The chosen points placed on your head, face, hands, arms, and legs will activate your whole body and send impulses to the sensory and motoric representation of your body in the brain. Your body representation is known as the Homunculus, or the "small man" or "small woman" in the brain. This mapping is your bodily blueprint for restoring a sense of your body's perfect integration and achieving a higher level of health. In a very short time, you will become aware of your heart and breathing, and you will be rooted in the present moment, experiencing a deep sense of calm and peace. Your troubled mind will not travel in the past or try to get a glimpse of the future. It will stay in the background, where it should be, to supervise your healing. Your breathing will shift from the stress-induced breathing located in your upper chest to the deep abdominal breath, well-oxygenating your relaxed body. Your deep breathing will continuously energize your **brain's meridian.** The 30 Needles Constellation Acupuncture and your new orbital breathing are among the best ways to connect with and deploy ancient wisdom, integrating it into your modern, health-oriented lifestyle.

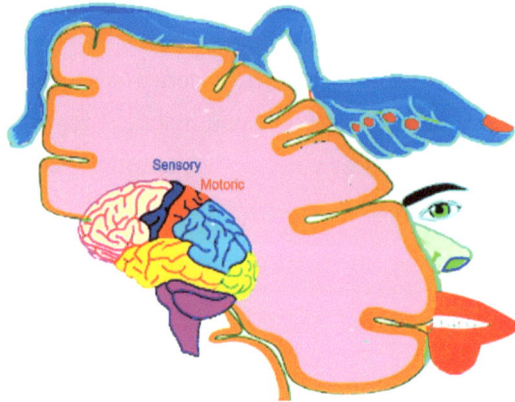

Picture 4. It depicts the Homunculus, the map of your body "small man" or "small woman" in your brain.

Two main energy vessels build your **brain's meridian**: the Governing and Conception Vessels. When this energetic duo is harmonized and balanced, it will contribute greatly to your physical vitality and intellectual clarity. Traditional medical practices such as Acupuncture, Qi Gong, Yoga, and Tai Chi focus on cultivating and intentionally accelerating the flow of vital energy in the brain meridian. These ancient treatment and exercise techniques emphasize the importance of balance in the front and rear parts of the brain meridian to achieve perfect health and a harmonious sense of well-feeling.

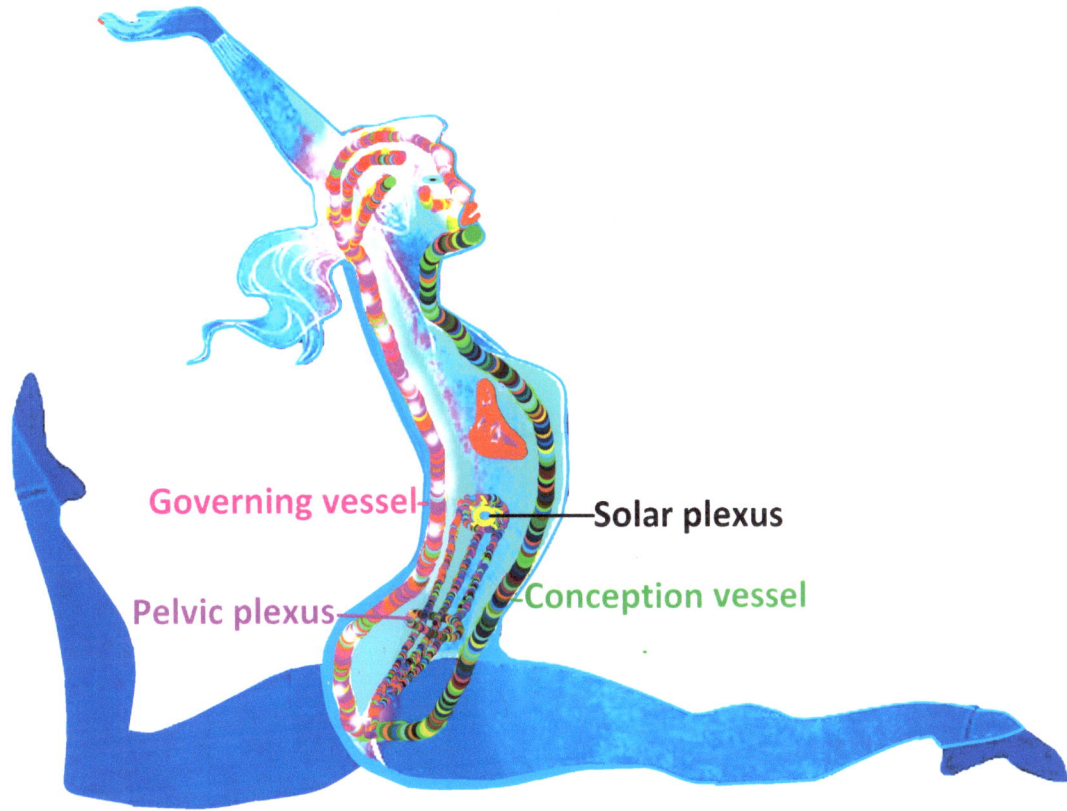

Picture 5. It displays the Conception and Governing Vessels building the brain meridian and its relation to the Solar- and Pelvic plexus.

The Governing and the Conception Vessels, as your **brain meridian**, are seen as the energetic key in traditional medicine to regulate your bodily energy at all times in the best possible balance between the forces of yin and yang. The back part of the brain meridian is the Governing Vessel. Its name comes from the pathway over the spinal cord in the back of your body, which governs muscles, skin, and supplies your internal organs.

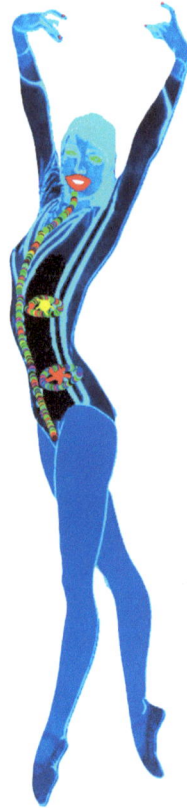

Picture 6. Conception Vessel and its relation to Solar and Pelvic plexus.

The front part of the brain meridian is named in traditional medicine as the Conception Vessel. Simplifying the complexity of your body, the front is designed for energy intake. In contrast, the back of your body governs the absorbed vital energy. It is rooted in ancient healing wisdom. The activated orbital breathing connects you to the energy source, which originates in the lower/middle abdomen, specifically within the Solar and Pelvic plexus. This space where the first impulse for your every breath originates is located inside your abdomen is known as the Chinese term Dantien. Dantien translates into English as "The Gate to Heaven".

The 30 needles inserted in your body in a special constellation target the energy channels and the functions of your internal organs, particularly your brain and heart. Your beating heart responds to the needles placed at the heart energy channel by increasing blood supply to itself first, and then to your brain. The invigorated heart will then increase blood supply to your kidneys, accelerating the detox process, and then to your gut, initiating the cleansing of your body.

Particularly noteworthy are the special mini molecular motors in your body, known as *kinases*. They will be activated by acupuncture. The *kinases* are the front-line workers inside of your body. Derived from the Greek word 'kinein', which means to move and to set in motion, they initiate the repair of your organs, and they give a kick-start for the replenishment of your energy. Every molecular motor inside your cells strives for perfection and operates at high speed.

They will also exchange the stagnant water and move the toxins to the outside of your body. Your body will speed up its metabolism, enhance muscle regeneration, and increase the release of stem cells.

After 30 minutes and the removal of the needles, you will feel refreshed, and your energy will be replenished. Your eyes will be wide open, and you will be aware of everything. You will become aware of your body feeling deeply connected to your spiritual self.

3

Acupuncture tradition and the modern view

If there is free flow, there is no pain; if there is pain, there is lack of free flow. **Huang Di Nei Jing.**

Traditional Chinese medicine identifies fourteen energy channels, which can be accessed through the use of acupuncture needles. Of these fourteen energy channels, half of them is classified as *"yang"*, indicating the flow of energy from top to bottom, metaphorically described as from "heaven to earth" or from head to feet.

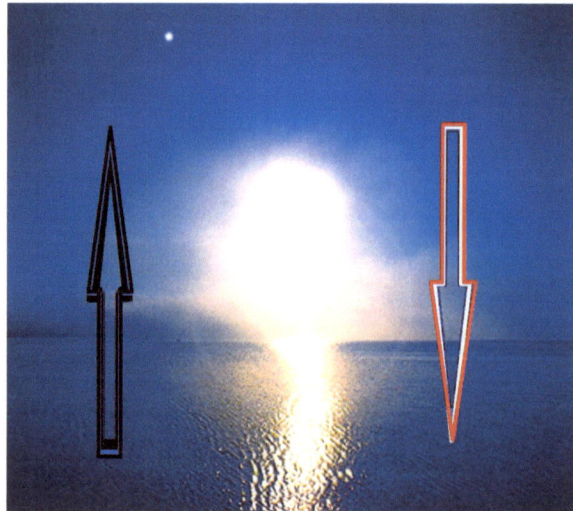

Picture 7. It is an illustration of the yin-yang forces.

Yang is associated with attributes such as activity, dynamism, governance, masculinity, movement, light, and fire. The remaining seven, termed as "*yin*" energy channels, are considered to ascend from the feet to the top of the head, or from "earth to heaven." Yin is characterized by passivity and receptivity, and is commonly associated with femininity, darkness, water, and earth. This symbolic framework contributes to a nuanced understanding of the balance of your bodily energy channels.

Acupuncture is a well-established medical intervention and has not developed overnight. It has a rich tradition of over 2000 years of successful treatment and healing.

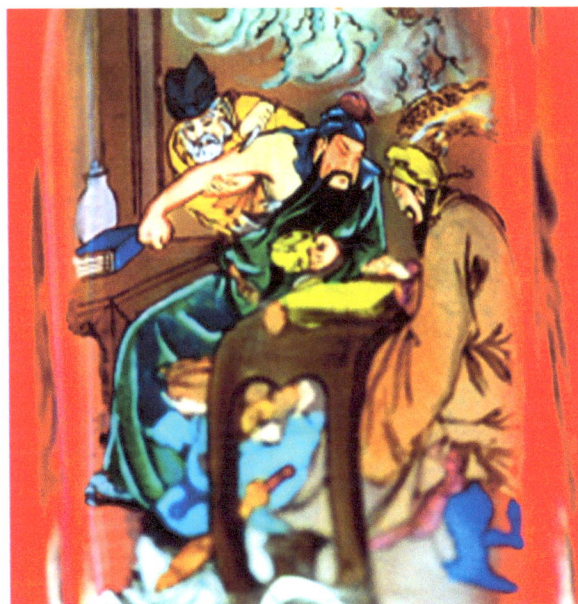

Picture 8. This is the image of Dr. Hua Tuo in his ancient clinical practice, painted by an unknown artist.

Dr. Hua Tuo, an outstanding Chinese acupuncturist, made significant contributions to the acupuncture framework. His influential legacy of the 48 acupuncture points along the spine is still being practiced world wide.

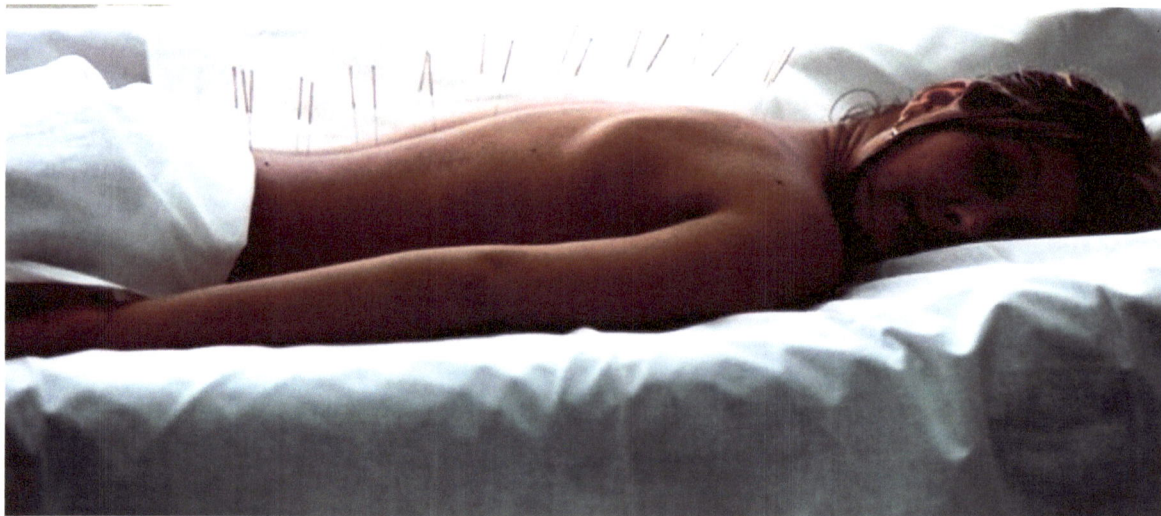

Picture 9. It is an illustration of an acupuncture treatment with the needles placed on Dr Hua Tuo's points alongside the spine.

China was home to four prominent acupuncture schools, each possessing a rich historical legacy before the establishment of Universities for Traditional Medicine in China in the 1960s. These schools, located in Beijing, Chengdu, Shanghai, and Guangdong, were the key centers for traditional Chinese acupuncture.

Each school has cultivated distinctive acupuncture techniques, many of which cannot be found in conventional textbooks. The core needle techniques, a key aspect of these healing methods, were traditionally transmitted orally. This means that the knowledge was typically shared only with trusted apprentices. The trust between teacher and student was of utmost importance, highlighting the personal nature in the field of medical acupuncture.

I completed my acupuncture training under Dr. Li Jian in 1991, 1992, and 1997 at Xuan-Wu Hospital, the teaching facility affiliated with the University of Traditional Chinese Medicine in Beijing. This mentorship with Dr. Li, a prominent member of the Beijing School of Acupuncture, was instrumental, leaving a deep imprint on my experiences of effective acupuncture treatments.

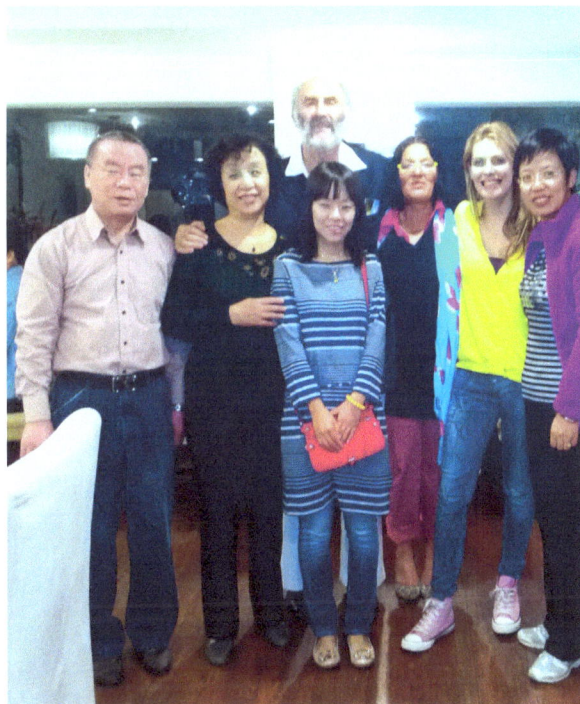

Picture 10. The image displays Dr Li and Dr George, with their families in Beijing in 2013. On the right is the Sunflower, our interpreter and friend.

Dr. Li's groundbreaking introduction of a constellation of 30 needles on specific acupuncture points marked a transformative moment in the integration of my modern and traditional medical knowledge. This traditional and innovative approach not only challenged me as an established medical doctor and specialist in internal medicine, deeply grounded in contemporary medical knowledge and research, but also opened new medical perspectives. Over time, I have observed that nearly all conditions I treated showed significant improvement and more often a spectacular healing effect. Throughout my acupuncture training, the 30 Needles Constellation Acupuncture consistently demonstrated remarkable efficacy. The practicality and versatility of medical acupuncture, along with its proven advantages across a broad spectrum of medical conditions I have encountered in my clinical work, have become increasingly evident to me. The continuously growing success of my acupuncture treatments reinforced my confidence and trust in the 30 Needles Constellation Acupuncture, establishing it as a cornerstone of my medical acupuncture practice.

The modern view on acupuncture.

From the perspective of 21st-century medical knowledge, acupuncture is recognized as a therapeutic procedure that works with the body's energy channels and specific acupuncture points to regulate the function of muscles, ligaments, bones, and the internal organs. The energy channels are closely linked with major sensory and motor nerves, forming connections between the brain, heart, and spinal cord. Critical centers such as the Solar plexus, which is responsible for breathing, your body's fight or flight response, and the pelvic Plexus, which regulates reproductive and digestive functions, play essential roles within this amazing network.

Communication between cells occurs through electromagnetic waves, similar to those used by antennas and mobile phones. The impulses are received by the nerve cells and then conducted to muscles and internal organs via electrical current. During acupuncture, sterile needles are inserted to stimulate specific points that act as gateways between the body's interior and the energy of the external fields. The acupuncture points are characterized by a great number of unique sensors and a rich blood vessel network, establishing direct links with the heart and brain. Acupuncture enhances the functionality of your body's self-organizing system. It plays a vital role in regulating the flow of energy to maintain perfect body balance, improving your bodily awareness, and calming your mind.

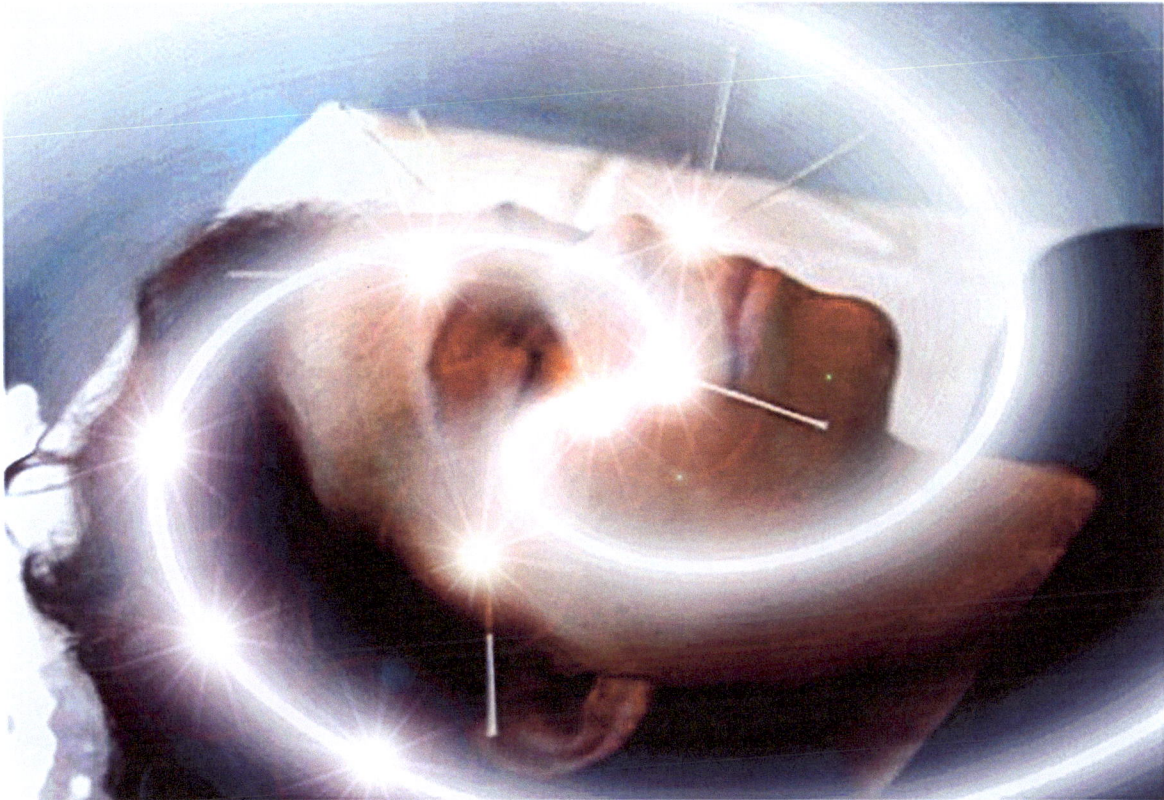

Picture 11. It is a modern artist's vision of the electromagnetic impact of acupuncture.

The entry points for needle insertion can adjust the movements of vital energy, responding dynamically to your body's needs. This process can accelerate or slow down physiological functions depending on your body's needs. In times of distress, acupuncture moderates the excess and intensity of energy flow, promoting balance through the functional adjustment of nerves, blood, lymph, and other bodily fluids.

Specifically, acupuncture activates molecular motors, known as *kinases*, to facilitate the cleansing process and create a clear pathway for your regeneration.

4

How acupuncture works

When modern science discovers how to go deep into the subtle electromagnetic constitution of man, it will be able to correct almost any medical condition in ways that would seem almost miraculous today. In the future, healing will be affected more and more by the use of various types of light rays. Light is what we are made of—not gross physical light, but the finer spiritualized light of prana, intelligent life energy. Paramahansa Yogananda.

30 Needles Constellation Acupuncture is a method for treating all functional medical conditions and promoting genuine healing. According to today's standards, it sometimes seems nearly miraculous.

Acupuncture works at many levels within your complex body. Remember, your body is a self-organizing system, and you must give it a chance to replenish vital energy and restore a healthy balance through acupuncture, rest, abdominal breathing, and your bodily awareness. All these actions initiated by acupuncture needles support your self-healing potential.

Network of energy channels of your body.

The design of the energy channels of your body is a fascinating network. There are fourteen energy channels, each with entry points that can be accessed with acupuncture needles. They are all connected to your brain, heart, and spinal cord. They are also linked to your solar plexus, a bundle of radiating nerve fibers located in the upper abdomen, just behind the stomach and the diaphragm. According to 21st-century research, your energy channels run alongside the major sensory and motoric nerves, forming a complex network that has direct connections to your brain and heart. The information between neurons is transmitted wirelessly by means of electromagnetic waves through structures on their surface, akin to antennas. These antennas collect your wireless commands from the brain and transmit the impulses to the inside of your cells.   Amazingly, you can, through your electromagnetic thoughts, voluntarily accelerate your breathing or initiate muscle relaxation. This is the evidence and confirmation that you have control over your body's energy system.

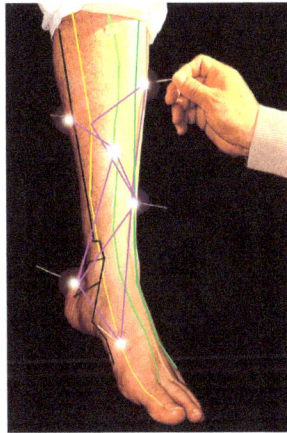

Picture 12. It illustrates the selected acupuncture points with energy channels forming a network on the leg.

The energy channels and acupuncture points form a fantastic network, as illustrated in the picture above. The hand performing the acupuncture is Dr. Li's, and the leg belongs to the author. The photo was taken on the train as we traveled to deliver the acupuncture lectures in Germany in summer of the year 2000.

A 30 Needles Constellation Acupuncture, combined with orbital breathing and expansion of your awareness, is the super-key to your healing.

The perfect outcome of your healing lies in combining orbital breathing with acupuncture on the energy channels, along with training your bodily awareness, as well as welcoming the negative thoughts. Acupuncture positively impacts your consciousness, helping you become more aware of your body and sense both your immediate and distant surroundings. Acupuncture and breathing keep you in the present moment. You can experience the absolute *now* rather than dwelling on thoughts about your past.

Sometimes negative thoughts that appear during your treatment can stem from various sources, including past experiences, particularly from your childhood, your parents, societal influences, and even your evolutionary background, known as the generational or "junk DNA". While treated with 30 Needles Constellation Acupuncture, learn to pay attention to the present moment and be without judgment or discrimination. It will allow you to observe negative thoughts as they arise. They are nothing but electromagnetic frequencies and vibrations. Be much like a neutral observer and do not touch them in any way, and they will dissolve. Imagine your negative thoughts as clouds passing in the sky or leaves floating down a stream. You are the observer, not the cloud or leaf.

Negative thoughts are stored in your subconscious mind. When you welcome them from an observer's perspective, it frees up more life energy, and you will feel pleasant relaxed, and re-energized. Suppressing negative thoughts comes at a high energetic expense. By leaving the internal turmoil of your thoughts untouched and simply being aware, you can redirect your energy toward the interior of your body. Once the negative cellular experiences you have had in the past reach the surface of your body during acupuncture treatment, they will be dissolved and never return.

Through heightened awareness of your body, gained through acupuncture and orbital breathing, you will be able to expand to the bigger picture of your apartment or home, your city, and beyond. Whenever you lie on the treatment table, in New York, Perth, known as the City of Light, Paris, London, New Delhi, Beijing, Munich, Warsaw, or Oberstdorf, your awareness will expand to all sides, encompassing rooms, buildings, churches, rivers, forests, seas, the ground, and the sky. You can see yourself from midair and realize the presence of the moon or sun, stars, and know that your own spaceship, the Earth, is traveling at a speed of 30 km per second.

Brain meridian, oxygen, and light for the self-organizing system of your body

The speed of your recovery and healing depends on the increased oxygenation of your brain and activation of your brain meridian.

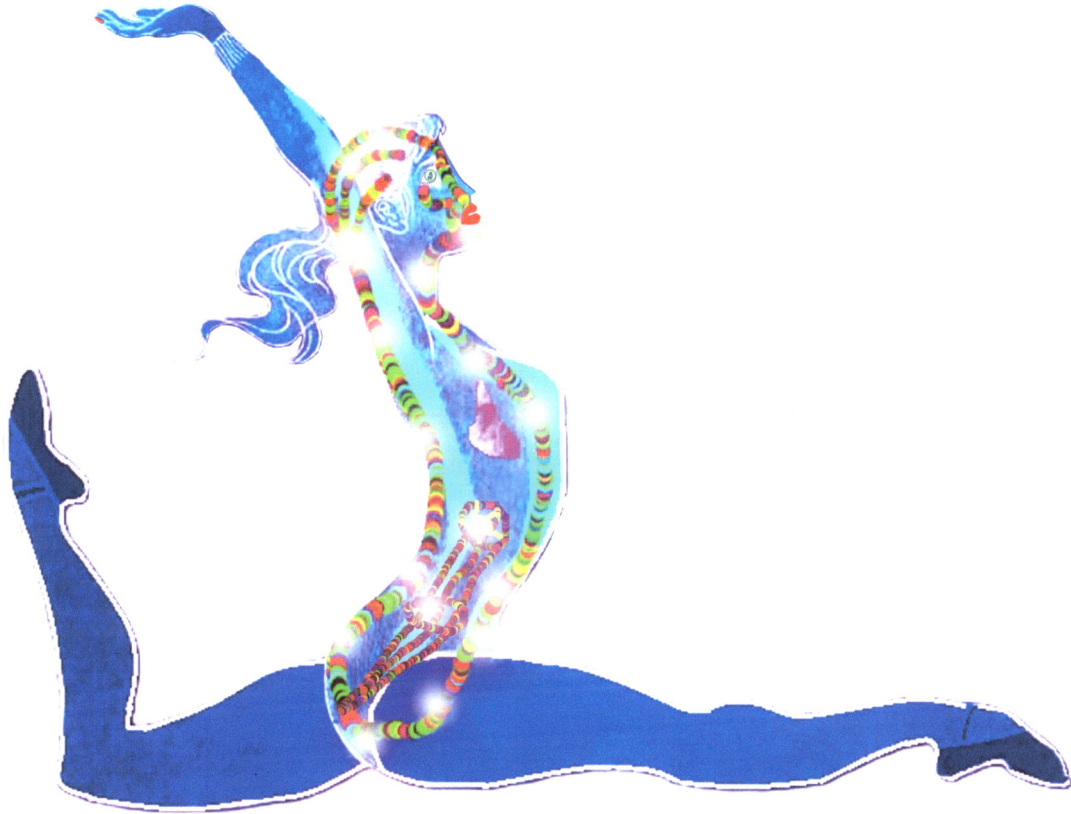

Picture 13. It displays the brain meridian and the flow of vital energy while you practice orbital breathing.

The balance of your energy channels and your ability to adapt flexibly to various types of light and frequencies, such as thoughts and electromagnetic fields, determine your recovery. Acupuncture needles interact with the body's field and the electromagnetic frequencies of light. It restores the body's self-organizing system and its full functionality. Light constitutes the essence of your being—not just the gross physical light visible to the eye, but the finer, spiritualized light known as the intelligent life energy.

The discovery of orbital breathing, where the flow of life energy accelerates alongside the brain meridian, is not just a revelation but a genuinely life-changing experience that will transform your understanding of health and wellness. Advances in medical science demonstrate that oxygen plays a dominant role in the body's self-organizing system by promoting tissue healing, reducing inflammation, and regulating cellular detox. Deep abdominal and orbital breathing increases your oxygen uptake. It promotes healing by stimulating white defense cells, growing new small vessels, and releasing stem cells. Light interacts with biological molecules to stimulate cellular functions, thereby enhancing tissue repair and aiding in conditions such as chronic inflammation and pain. The brain plasticity will increase and you will continuously learning new things and patterns in your new lifestyle. Your brain has a remarkable ability to generate daily patterns that control rhythms such as breathing, digesting food, and walking.

Recent research from Japan on energy channels, a framework in traditional Chinese medicine, has provided new evidence since 2017. Meridians or energy channels may exist as a " neurological map" in specific parts of the brain, not as physical structures like blood vessels or nerves. This finding is part of a growing body of research that uses modern magnetic resonance imaging MRI to explore the neurological basis of acupuncture and meridians.

Recent research from Japan and other countries suggests that meridians, the energy pathways in the body, may exist in the brain not as a physical structure, but as a ' neuro-mapping' network within the nervous system. This network, a functional pathway possibly through the central nerve pathways, fascial tissue, and connective tissue matrix, can be visualized and quantified using modern imaging techniques like functional magnetic resonance imaging fMRI. These findings could have significant implications for integrative health, offering new avenues for your acupuncture treatment and very important for your effective awareness training.

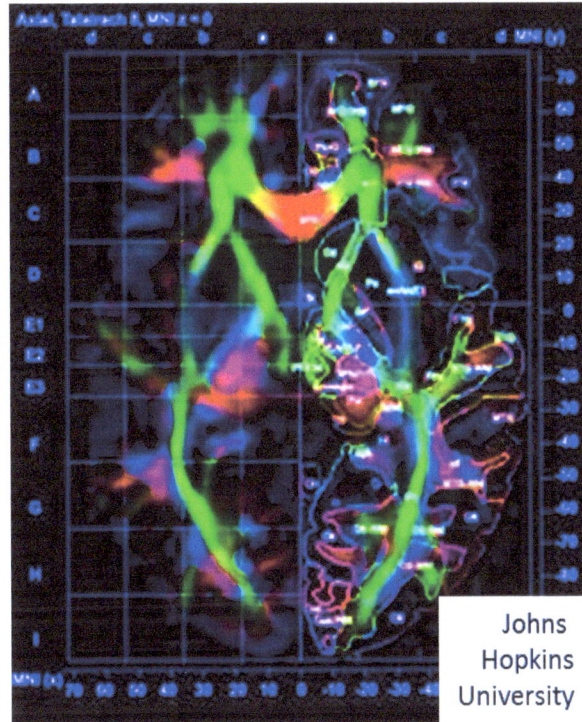

Picture 14. It is depicting a section through the diffusion weighted MRI of a brain. Section generated at Johns Hopkins University on 19 January 2016. Author Mim.cis. Own work. Wikipedia.

These findings could revolutionize our understanding of the energy channels and their neuronal foundation, opening up new approach for research and treatment. Modern science has made remarkable discoveries regarding the subtle electromagnetic constitution of the human body and the nature of cellular breathing. The researchers gained the ability to explore the most delicate energetic structures of the human body.

5

30 Needles Constellation Acupuncture

When Jesus died on the cross and cried out "It is finished", He not only died for our sins, but also for our diseases, too. Kathryn Kuhlman.

The **30 Needles Constellation Acupuncture** is characterized by the precision of its 30 carefully selected points, which are applied symmetrically on both sides of the body, along with a few single extra-points. The 30 Needles Constellation Acupuncture needles target the following organs and bodily functions.

- *Stage one* consists of insertion of **12 needles** in the acupuncture points at your head and face. They target your brain and its Homunculus. The first needle will be inserted at the acupuncture point GV20-Baihui of the brain meridian, the following four needles will be placed around the top of the head at the extra-point SiShenCong. Additional two needles will be inserted bilateral at the extra-point Taiyang on your temples. The next 2 needles will be placed at the acupuncture points LI20, Yingxiang, at the cheeks beside the nose of the large intestine energy channel. Last single needle will be placed at the acupuncture point Shuigou, GV26, above the upper lip of the brain meridian,

- *Stage two* includes the insertion of **8** needles. They are dedicated to your hands and forearms. They are targeting the improvement of your Intelligent Heart, your lungs, and all organs, which are situated in your chest. Your heart and lungs are vital organs that require special attention during this treatment. First two needles will be be inserted bilaterally at the acupuncture point H7, Shenmen of the heart energy channel. Two more needles will be inserted at the acupuncture point L7, Lieque of the lung energy channel, 4 cm above the wrist. Another two needles, will be placed bilaterally at the LI4, Hegu, acupuncture point of the large intestine energy channel, between the thumb and index finger, and two last needles at the acupuncture points LI11, Quchi, on both elbows also of the large intestine energy channel. These needles at the points of the large intestine channel target the improvement of your immune system and the blood supplay to your skin, brain and face.

- *Stage three* encompass the placement **10 needles.** They will be inserted in your legs to replenish the functionality of all internal organs, which are situated in the abdomen. These needles target also all your tendons, ligaments holding your spine and shaping your face. It is important to note that one needle will be inserted bilaterally at the acupuncture point ST36, Zusanli, of the stomach energy channel. The ST36 point is located on the side of your calf, 5 cm under the knee cap. Two more needles will be placed at the acupuncture points GB34 Yuanlinquan of the gall bladder energy channel, on the side of the calf, about 3 cm below the side bone of the knee, and another two needles at the acupuncture points SP6, Sanyinjiao of the spleen energy channel, approximately 5 cm above each inner ankle bone. Similarly, two needles will be inserted bilaterally at the acupuncture point K3, Taixi of the kidney energy channel, one needle in each ankle, in the middle between the inside ankle bone and Achilles tendon, and two last needles, one on each foot between the big toe and the second toe at the acupuncture point LIV3, Taichong of the liver energy channel.

Benefits and Methodology

30 Needles Constellation Acupuncture is designed to enhance your overall vitality, reduce stress load on your heart, and initiate your body's self-healing. The technique consists of inserting needles in pairs on both the left and right sides for symmetrical acupuncture points, such as H7 of the heart

energy channel, which requires one needle in each wrist and a inserting a single needle for specific extra point locations, like GV26 above your upper lip.

How It Works

By combining bilateral points at your energy channels and a single and bilateral extra-points, this acupuncture constellation supports the body's self-organizing capacity to respond strongly to the stimulation from the inserted acupuncture needles. 30 Needles Constellation Acupuncture is particularly beneficial for heart and brain health, and it also accelerates liver detoxification, resulting in a profound feeling of rejuvenation. Additionally, it supports better digestion and immune system, stimulating your cells to exchange the stagnant water and to enhance their cellular breathing. 30 Needles Constellation Acupuncture also resets the genetic messenger RNA (mRNA) to its normal activity.

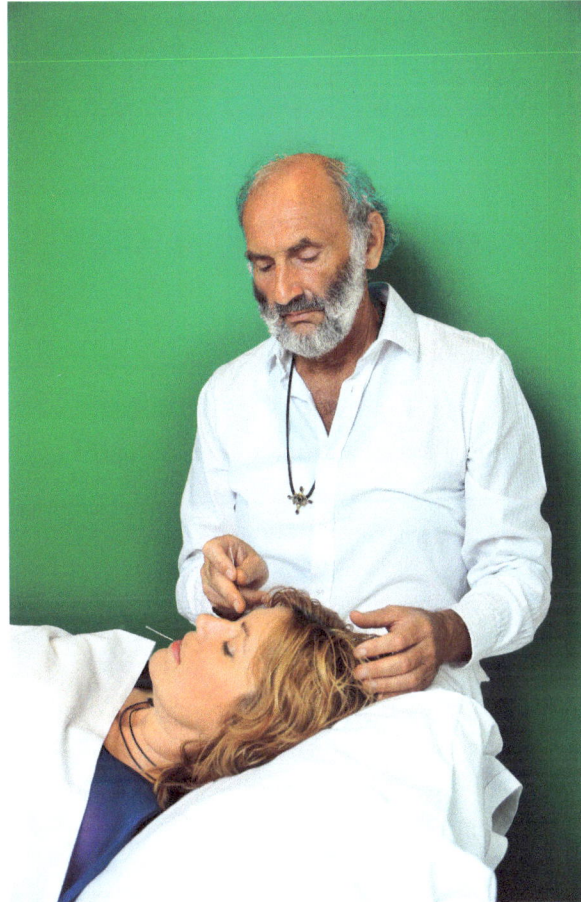

**Picture 15. It illustrates how Dr. George begins the
treatment with the 30 Needles Constellation Acupuncture
in a clinical setting.**

As a result, 30 needles Constellation Acupuncture while supporting the heart, brain, liver, and immune system, will leave you feeling cleansed, revitalized, and better equipped to handle the future stress load on your heart.

In this clinical illustration of an acupuncture treatment, Dr. George has already inserted needles at the Yingxiang point, located at the cheek beside the nose. Yingxiang, in translation to English, means "Welcome Fragrances." It is the twentieth acupuncture point of the large intestine energy channel, LI20. He is preparing to place an acupuncture needle at the second acupuncture point of the urinary bladder channel UB2, located just above the eyebrow, known as Zhanzhu, which translates in English to "Young Bamboo Bunch." This name arises from observations that sometimes needling at this site can rapidly elevate the point and surrounding tissues, reminiscent of the swift growth of young bamboo shoots.

In summary, the 30 Needles Constellation Acupuncture technically consists of three stages of acupuncture treatment.

- *Stage one* includes the insertion of 12 needles for your head and face, which is the first part of your treatment.
- *Stage two* involves the insertion of eight needles into your hands and forearm, which is the second important part of your acupuncture treatment.
- *Stage three* encompasses the placement of 10 needles in your legs, which accomplishes the 30 Needles Constellation Acupuncture.

The time of treatment is usually 30 minutes after the placement of the acupuncture needles is finished. The following chapters describe the practical application of the 30 Needles Constellation Acupuncture, detailing the insertion of each needle one by one.

6

The first stage of the acupuncture treatment

Repeated performance of an action creates a mental blueprint, causing the formation of the subtle electrical pathway in the brain-somewhat like a grooves in a phonograph record. Paramahansa Yogananda.

Most of my patients initially exhibited disturbed and unnatural breathing, primarily originating from the upper chest. The key indicator of correct abdominal breathing, the movement of the belly expanding with each inhalation, was absent in almost all of them. Many struggled to understand when I encouraged them to engage their belly. Recognizing the importance of this, I have included abdominal breathing into my acupuncture practice.

It has been a surprising revelation. To my greatest astonishment, I observed that inserting the acupuncture needles on the head and the face, in the extra-point ShiShenCong, extra-point Taiyang, UB2 points of the urinary bladder channel, GV20, and especially the needle at the point GV26, both of the brain meridian, visibly unlocked the deep abdominal, diaphragmatic breathing. What was even more striking was the emotional release that followed the return of normal, abdominal breathing. Many patients started to cry, while some were laughing intensely, and the tension in their bodies was released. This aspect of the 30 Needles Constellation Acupuncture is a powerful support for emotional healing.

Encouraged by the excellent healing capacity of Swedish Bitters, which I experienced with my wonderful wife, Angela, during our honeymoon in Athens and at the Acropolis, the birthplace of Western civilization, I started to apply Swedish Bitters topically to my patients. I placed the facial tissues soaked with Swedish Bitter on their foreheads, arms and legs, sometimes even covered their eyes with it. To my utmost delight, they loved it too; they appreciated the smell and fragrances of the tincture, as well as its soothing and calming effects.

Swedish Biters originates from a recipe developed by the 16th-century physician Paracelsus, who called his version *Elixir ad longam vitam*, in translation, the medicine for a long life. This potent formulation of herbs prepared as a tincture was rediscovered in the 18th century by Swedish physician Dr. Claus Samst. Doctor Samst recorded his version of the formula and used it for various ailments before his death. The Swedish doctor also wrote a manuscript describing the 43 conditions for which Swedish Bitters can bring relief. Dr Samst himself lived to be 104 and finally fell asleep, not because of old age, but as a result of a fall and its complications while out riding a horse.

Swedish Bitters was brought to public attention by the Austrian herbalist Maria Treben. Her book, *Health Through God's Pharmacy*, popularized the remedy, which is based on an ancient elixir and contains a blend of bitter herbs. Swedish bitters are a traditional herbal remedy primarily used to support the digestive system. They are beneficial for your heart by stimulating cardiac function and normalizing the lipid profile.

When applied topically, as I do with the 30 Needles Constellation Acupuncture, it acts as an antiallergic and antiseptic. It also increases the blood supply to the area of application. When asked about Swedish Bitters, I recommend applying it topically for skin irritations, minor wounds, bruises, and to reduce tissue swelling.

The 30 Needles Constellation Acupuncture, a cornerstone of my practice, is designed to restore the body's energy flow, correct breathing patterns, and promote calmness in your mind. It achieves this by stimulating the body's representation in the brain, the Homunculus. The procedure begins with the placement of 12 needles at the head and face, **with the first needle** at the pivotal acupuncture point GV20 Baihui, at the top of your head, of the brain meridian, which is marked with light.

It is imperative to align the direction of the acupuncture needles at the point GV20 with the vital energy flow during the inhalation phase of orbital breathing, from the crotch alongside your spine and the back of your head, and then down to the upper lip. The angle between the acupuncture needle and the surface of the head is less than 90 degrees. Otherwise, all the positive aspects of acupuncture could be diminished.

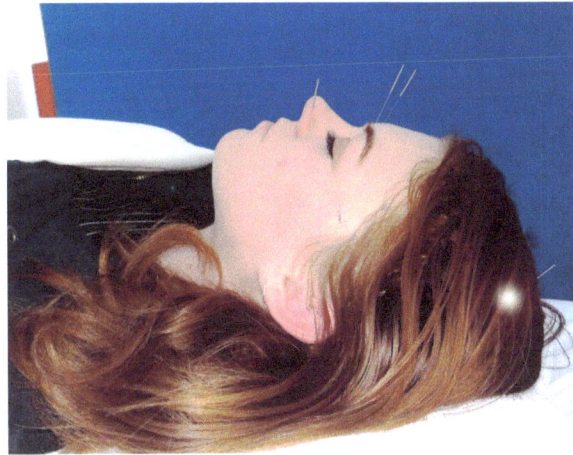

Picture 16. It illustrates a needle at the pivotal acupuncture point GV20 Baihui, located at the top of the head on the brain meridian.

The name Baihui of this special acupuncture point, when translated into English, means "Hundred Convergences" because it is a crucial meeting point for many of your body's energy channels. The activation of the GV20 with an acupuncture needle plays a role in stress regulation. It promotes the release of Cortisol, often referred to as an anti-stress hormone. The adrenal glands release Cortisol in response to stress, a vital component of your body's defense system. But Cortisol's influence extends beyond stress management. It is a chief hormone for most cells in your body, regulating metabolism, immune system strength, blood sugar levels, blood pressure, and even contributing to a good memory. The stimulation of the point GV20-Baihui restores your DNA blueprint and corrects the functioning of your mRNA, the messenger RNA. It plays a dominant role in the transfer of information within your body via messenger RNA, and how your body responds to viral infections.

Four needles, numbered 2, 3, 4, and 5, are strategically placed at the extra-point ShiShenCong, located around the top of the head. The Chinese term 'SiShenCong' translates to 'God's Cleverness' in English, reflecting its ability to calm the spirit, pacify the mind, and tranquilize any storm caused by external influences. This calming effect leaves you feeling relaxed and at ease.

Acupuncture point ShiShenCong regulates the brain functions, including memory, blood pressure regulation, and activation of the blue matrix for the self-organizing system of your body. It acts through the "small woman" or "small man" to be found in your brain, the Homunculus.

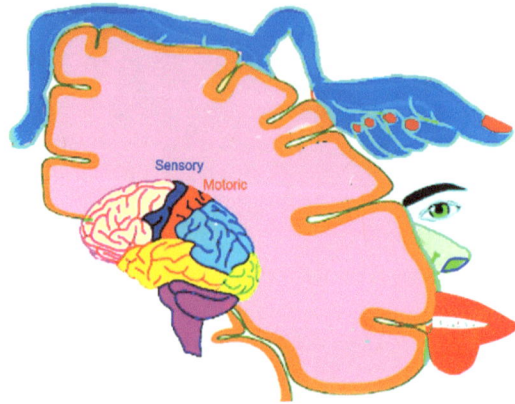

Picture 17. It displays the Homunculus, a "neurological map"illustrating how different regions of your brain correspond to specific motor and sensory functions throughout your body.

The Homunculus is essentially a "neurological map" that illustrates how different regions of your brain correspond to specific motor and sensory functions throughout your body. It is a specific brain area that influences very distinct motoric functions of your muscles and the sensitivity of your skin. It regulates the whole awareness and perception of your body,

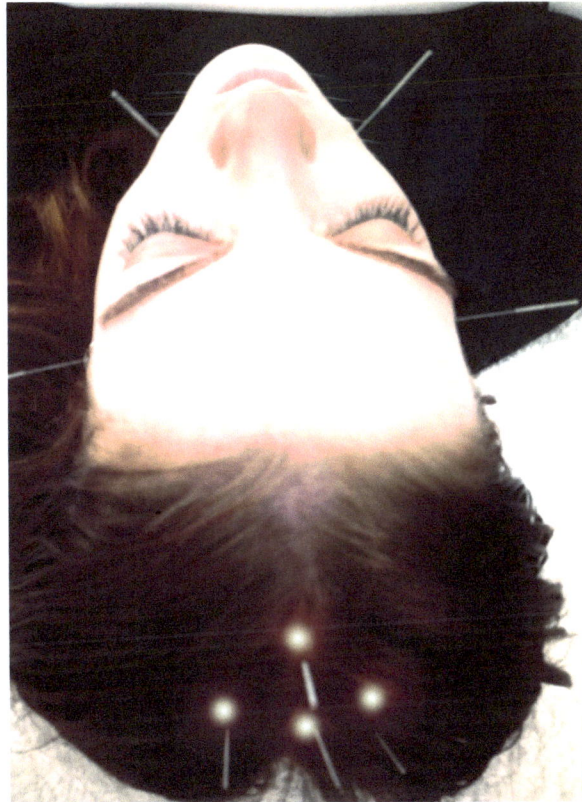

**Picture 18. This picture displays the acupuncture on the
extra-point ShiShenCong with inserted needles.**

Sometimes, it is fascinating to observe the responce to the insertion of **the needles 6 and 7** at the points UB2 of the urinary bladder energy channel, also known as Zhansu, which translates to "Bamboo Bunch" in English. They are inserted just above your eyebrows, a location that is important for the effectiveness of the treatment. Activation of the UB2 points is a comforting moment of acupuncture. When the acupuncture needles activate the point UB2, the energy stagnation caused by pollen or chemical allergy is released. The rapid swelling of the surrounding tissues, like the growth of young bamboo, signifies the instant release of stagnant vital energy. After a few minutes of acupuncture, the swelling decreases, and the skin returns to normal, marking a restored energy flow. The acupuncture at these points also corrects your intense eye use, providing good relief.

Acupuncture on the UB2 point is comforting for headaches, redness of the eyes, swollen eyes, eye pain, eyelid twitching, and cataracts.

Needles 8 and 9 are inserted at the extra-points Taiyang, located on both sides of the temples at the end of the eye arch. The Chinese term 'Taiyang' translates to 'The Sun' in English. Activation of this point not only enhances light uptake through the eyes but also has the potential to lower high blood pressure, making it a versatile acupuncture point in treating cardiovascular conditions.

Then, needles 10 and 11 are placed at the cheeks on both sides of the nose at the acupuncture point LI20, Yingxiang, of the large intestine energy channel. They target the normalization of breathing. The Chinese name Yingxiang, meaning "Welcome fragrances," adds a unique cultural dimension to the functionality of this acupuncture point, connecting you to the rich history of traditional Chinese medicine. The needles at the points LI20 on both sides of the nose facilitate effective breathing and improve discrimination in smelling. The LI20 Yingxiang acupuncture point is also the central point for the dysfunctions of your nose and your sensibility in sensing of fragrances.

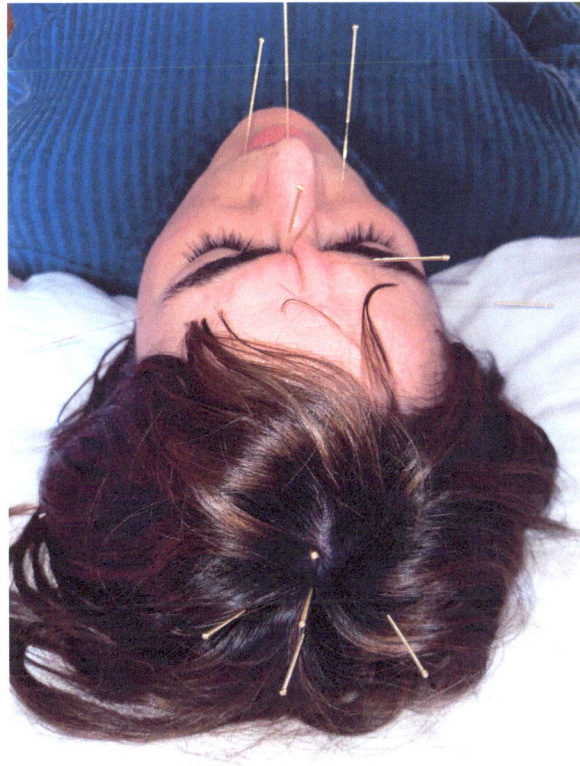

Picture 19. It displays the first stage of the 30 Needles Constellation Acupuncture with all 12 needles inserted in the face and head.

Then, **the last single needle, number 12, accomplishes** the first stage of the 30 Needles Constellation Acupuncture. The needle GV26 point is to be placed above the upper lip at the acupuncture point GV26 of your brain meridian. The point GV26, Shuigou, after translation into English, is "The Centre" of the brain meridian, which runs from the crotch alongside your entire spine, the midline of your head to end at the upper lip, and descends via the front midline of your body to the crotch.

The first stage of 30 Needles Constellation Acupuncture, consisting of 12 needles, includes the acupuncture point GV26. It activates the function of your brain and opens your breathing, which may have been blocked during a trauma or accident in the past and has persisted for a long time.

In the following Chapter 7 contains the description of the second stage of the 30 Needles Constellation Acupuncture, the placement of 8 needles addressing important acupuncture points on your hands and forearms.

7

The second stage of the acupuncture treatment

God made you in His image, and in this image lie all the beautiful qualities of Spirit. Paramahansa Yogananda.

The second stage of the 30 Needles Constellation Acupuncture includes 8 needles addressing points at your hands and forearms.

The needles 13 and 14 of the 30 Needles Constellation Acupuncture are placed in the seventh acupuncture point H7 of the heart energy channel on both wrists.

The heart energy channel is considered by traditional medicine to be the master key to the body's energetic system. Shen is the spiritual force residing in your heart. It is also the source of virtue, creativity, and health. According to traditional Chinese medicine, the heart channel originates from the heart in the chest and creates a network throughout your body. Two internal branches extend from the heart: one goes upwards to the tongue, eyes, and brain, while another goes downwards to the Solar plexus. The heart channel breaks through the middle of the armpit to outside of your body and continues along the arm to its last point at the tip of the small finger. It contains nine entry points.

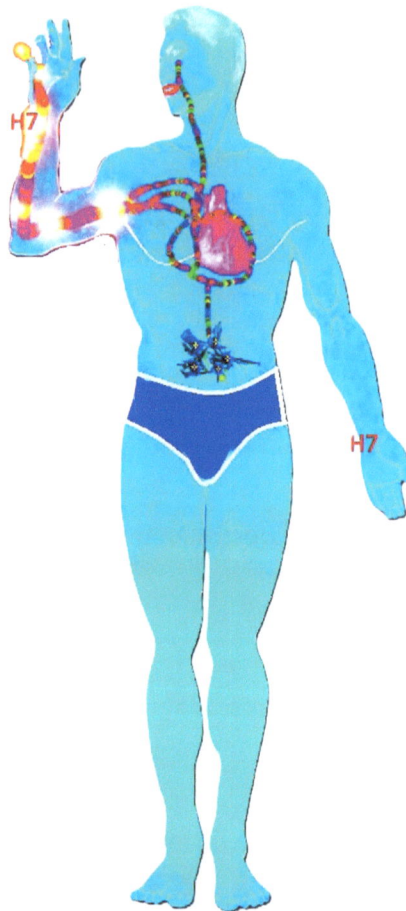

Picture 20. It displays the location of the acupuncture point H7, Shenmen on the heart energy channel.

Acupuncture at the H7 point improves sleep patterns and addresses insomnia. Furthermore, it reduces anxiety and promotes calmness, and most importantly, it supports a balance between your heart, soul, mind, body, and spirit.

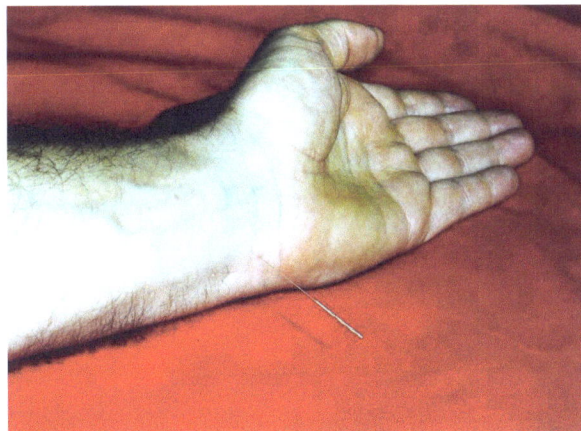

**Picture 21. A needle inserted in the acupuncture point
H7 of the heart energy channel.**

Needles number 15 and 16, which target the lungs, are inserted bilateral at the L7 acupuncture point of the lung energy channel. L7 point is also known as Lieque. The L7 acupuncture point Lieque translates into English "To Be Aligned". When the lungs are harmoniously aligned with the beating heart during breathing, their perfect cooperation will allow you to achieve your best bodily performance and achieve spiritual perception that transcends the ordinary three-dimensional world.

One internal branch of the lung energy channel extends upwards toward the throat and upper airways, and other internal branches connect with the lungs and heart. Another internal branch extends downwards to the Solar plexus. The lung energy channel internal branches connect also with the throat, lungs and heart linking the function of these organs 24/7 in an efficient and vigorous network.

The external lung energy channel originates below the collarbone to the thumb, comprising 11 acupuncture points. Notably, the seventh point of the lung energy channel, L7, is the master point for enhancing the function of all organs within the chest. Activating L7 points with acupuncture needles let your lungs fully engage with your whole energy network, allowing you deeper, more effective breathing. It improves the oxygenation of your lungs too. It is an initiation of lung healing by linking the lungs to the potential of your Intelligent Heart.

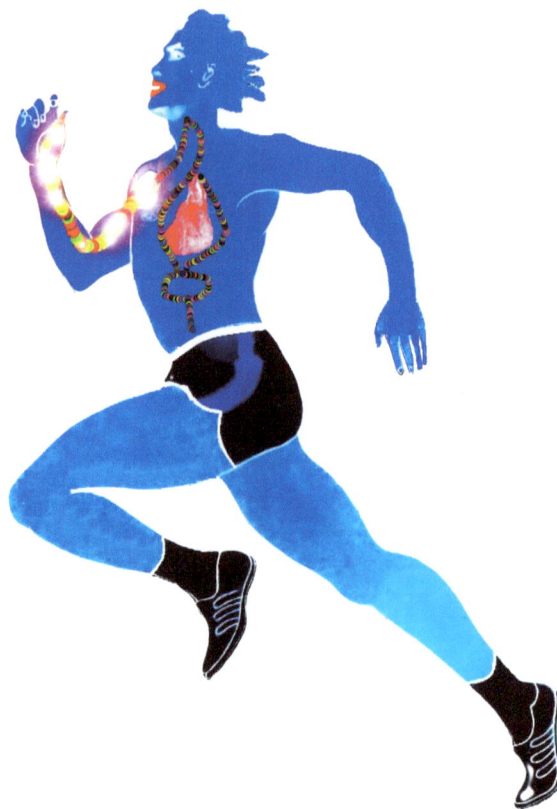

Picture 22. It displays the course of the lung energy channel.

The energy channel of the lung, in a funny language, "looks through the nose". It has an essential diagnostic meaning in cases of nasal congestion, rhinitis, and other early stages of upper airway dysfunction. The nose is affected first, but underlying this is the weakening of the lungs, which cannot deliver the appropriate amount of oxygen and energy during breathing.

Each human, including you and me, has two lungs. Your lungs do a vital job, performing about 15,000 breaths every day. They bring almost 9000 liters of air into your lungs. The air you breathe contains several gases, but you mainly need oxygen. With each breath, your lungs add fresh oxygen to your blood, which then carries it to the cells. On the way back, the blood brings out the toxins and carbon dioxide, which you expel. The primary function of your lungs is not just to supply the body with oxygen, but also to perform a crucial detoxification process. Therefore, it is important to use abdominal breathing using the diaphragm to extend the lungs to their full capacity maximizing the oxygenation and detox.

Each of your abdominal-based breaths brings us a volume of 300 to 400ml, in contrast to the chest type of breathing, also called 'stress breathing'. This type of breathing, often associated with shallow and rapid breaths, is a common response to stress or anxiety. It delivers only half of the volume of air into your lungs compared to abdominal breathing. The longer use of "stress breathing" can lead to decreased oxygenation and increased tension in your body.

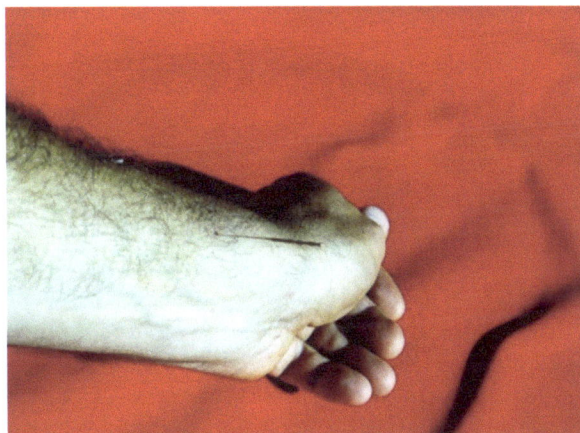

**Picture 23. It displays a needle inserted at the
acupuncture point L7 of the lung energy channel.**

The average involuntary frequency of your breathing mechanism is 6 to 8 breaths per minute.
You can increase your minute breath volume to 4 to five liters per minute. If you use your will, you can achieve much more. Please imagine that there are no limits in this area. The Olympic athletes used to ventilate 200 liters per minute. Some elite athletes, through their endurance training, breathe up to 6000 liters of air every hour while exercising. This illustrates to you the incredible po-

tential of your body to improve its breathing capacity with the right training and proven, safe techniques.

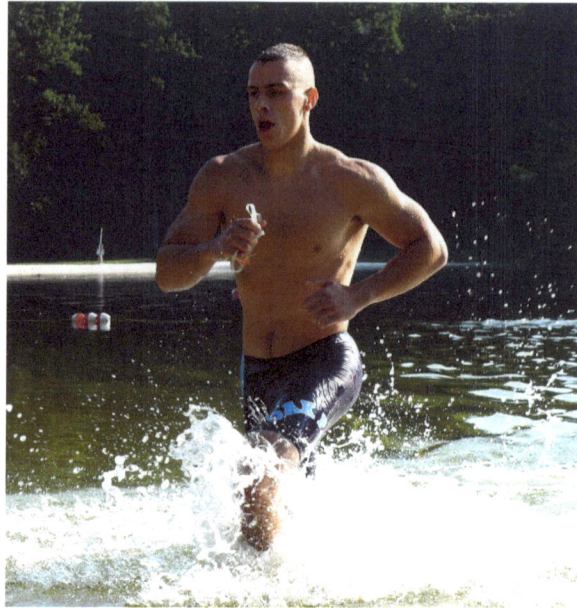

Picture 24. Lance Corporal Anthony M. Madonia emerges from the water during the swimming portion of the triathlon. Marines and Sailors of Marine Security Company and the Naval Support Facility in Thurmont, Maryland, participated in the Catoctin Mountain Triathlon Credit: Cpl. Earnest J. Barnes, Public domain, via Wikimedia Commons.

The lungs and large intestine perform similar main detox functions. The large intestine is the part of your body where the most water intake occurs. The large intestine is responsible for the absorption of water and the excretion of solid waste material. Food and waste material are moved along the length of your intestine by rhythmic contractions of intestinal muscles known as the peristaltic movements.

A very illustrative example of the functional connection between both organs and their mutual influence is the inflammatory process in the sinuses, which is very common. It's important to note that each of us, including you, experiences this kind of inflammatory response in the sinuses many times in a lifetime. This reassures us that such experiences are a normal part of our health journey.

The root cause lies in the large intestine, which does not absorb enough water and send it to the cells. Then the cells of the respiratory tract produce thickened mucus. It affects mainly the sinuses. Thick mucus cannot be removed easily and becomes fertile ground for bacterial growth.

Interestingly, the large intestine energy channel ends beside the nose at the twentieth point, LI20 and the acupuncture on it improves both lung and bowel function and is important for healing the inflammation in your sinuses.

The needles 17 and 18 of the 30 Needles Constellation Acupuncture are two needles inserted in the acupuncture points LI4-Hegu of the large intestine energy channel on both hands of the body, in the valley between the thumb and index finger. The large intestine channel is part of the 14 energy channels that have acupuncture points accessible for needle insertion.

The LI4 acupuncture point, or Hegu, has the meaning 'Union Valley' in English, is located between the extended thumb and index finger. It represents the union between men and women, as well as their social interactions. LI4 is vital for pain relief, as its stimulation releases Oxytocin, promoting feelings of well-being and fostering social bonding, trust, and empathy.

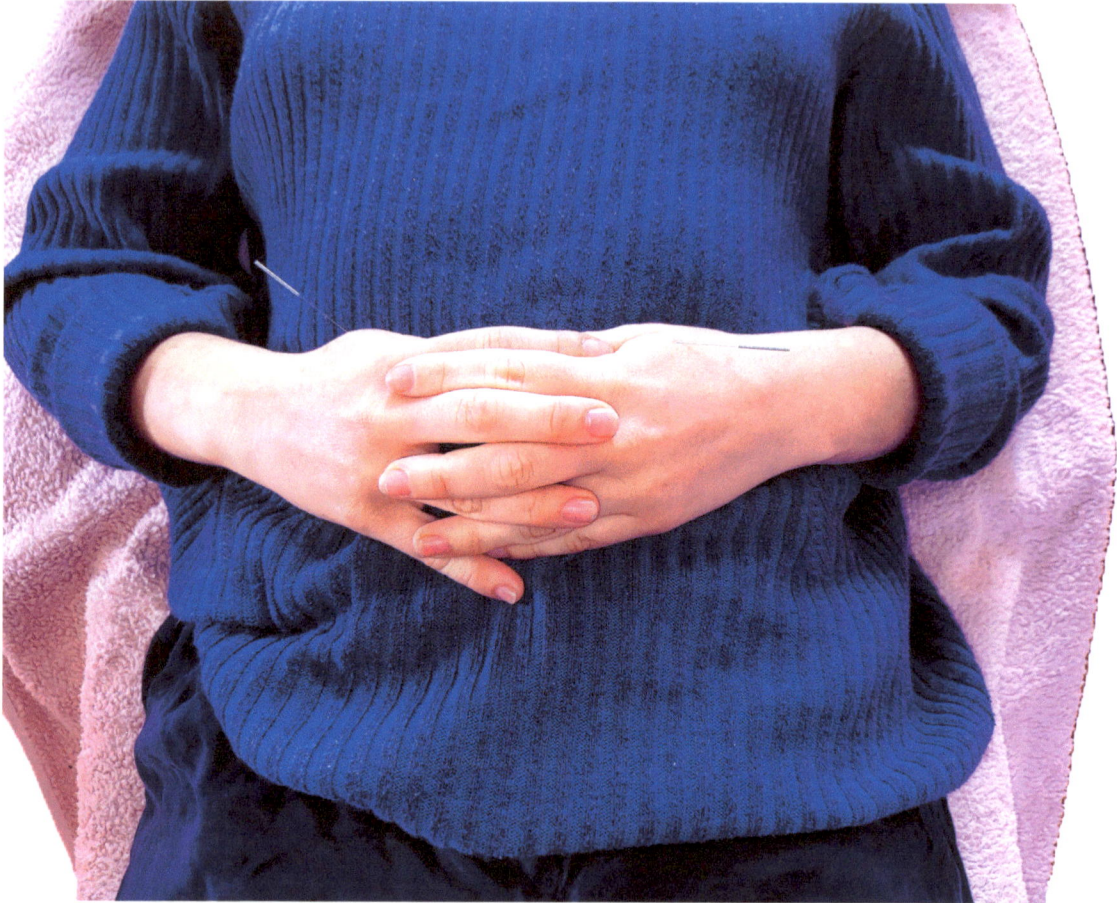

Picture 25. Acupuncture needles are inserted at the acupuncture points LI4 Hegu of the large intestine energy channel.

Oxytocin also induces uterine contractions, playing a vital role in childbirth, so extreme caution should be exercised when using the LI4 acupuncture point during pregnancy, especially before 37 weeks since conception.

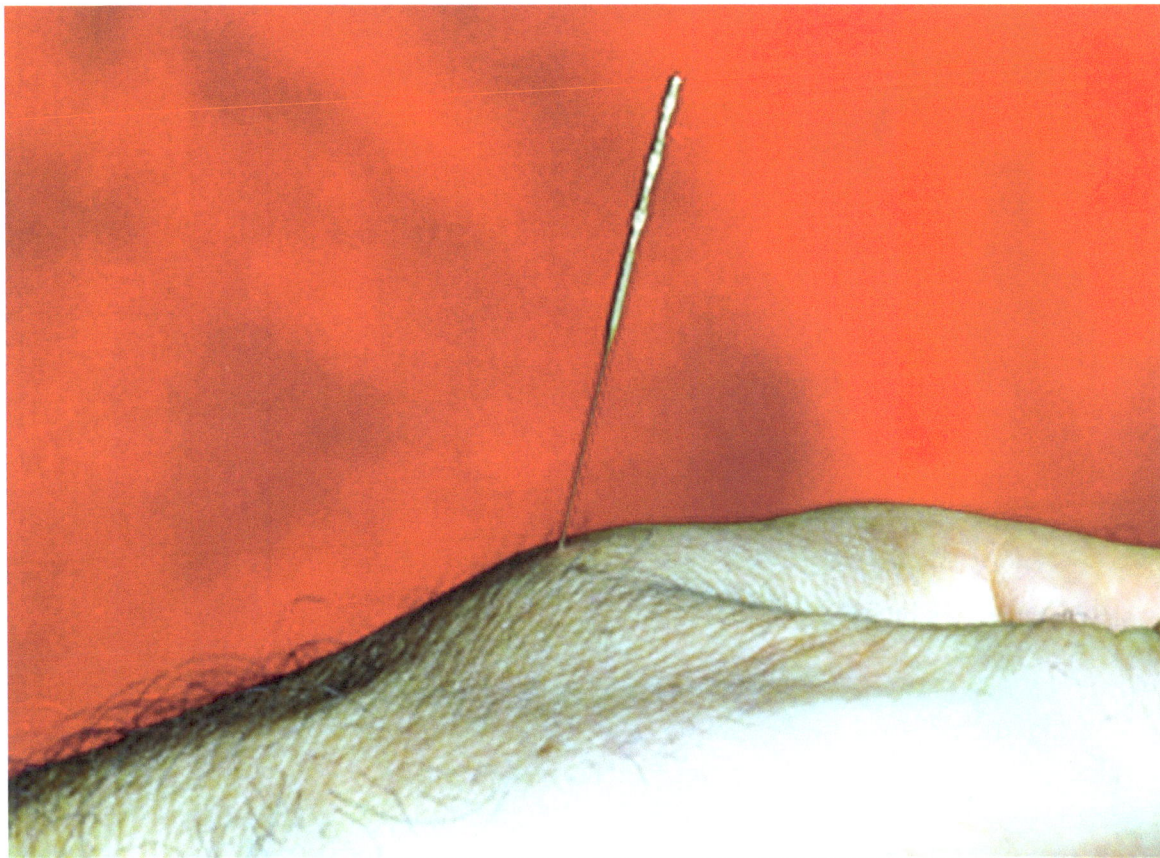

Picture 26. A needle is inserted at the acupuncture point LI4 Hegu of the large intestine energy channel.

Activation of the points LI4 also supports the peristalsis, the healthy gut movements. LI4 point of the large intestine energy channel is a Command point for the muscles and tendons of your face, mouth, teeth, and neck. The large intestine channel is part of the 14 energy channels that have acupuncture points accessible for needle insertion.

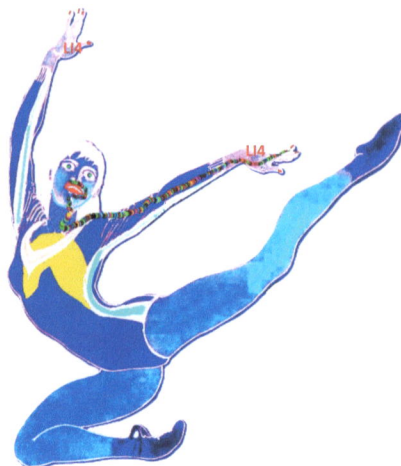

Picture 27. It displays the energy channel of the large intestine. Point LI4 is located on the hand in the valley between the thumb and index finger.

The LI4 point of the large intestine energy channel is a commonly used acupuncture point worldwide for its remarkable ability to effectively relieve pain and headaches. When the brain, gut, and heart work in harmony, it yields a range of benefits for the brain, digestive tract, and immune system.

Exciting contemporary research shows a link between Oxytocin and early childhood trauma, suggesting that the point LI4 can be stimulated to release the traumatic experiences you may have experienced as a small child.

The insertion of needles 19 and 20 is a fascinating process. For the person with very sensitive skin, the insertion of the needle at this point reduces skin sensitivity, allowing acupuncture to be continued with less or no pain at all. Acupuncture point LI11, also known as Quchi, in translation to English it means "The Pond of Vital Energy at the Bend," is located on the large intestine energy channel. These points possess a remarkable ability to act as a "cooling breeze", effectively cooling down inflammatory and allergic responses. This unique "cooling effect " of any inflammation is a key aspect of the role of the LI11 points in 30 Needles Constellation Acupuncture treatment. The activation of these points addresses your skin and gut, two largest organs of your body.

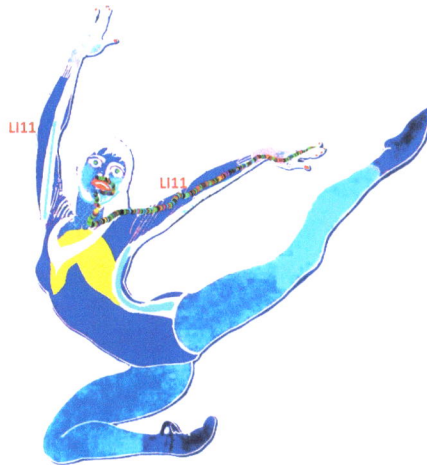

Picture 28. The large intestine energy channel course features the marked acupuncture points LI11, known as Quchi.

LI11 point is positioned at the end of the crease of the elbow; they are recognized for their effectiveness in clearing the skin, reducing inflammation, and regulating both the immune and digestive systems. The inserted needles at points LI11 help soothe a sore throat, reduce toothache, and relieve abdominal cramps. Their frequent use is justified in addressing musculoskeletal pain, immune response issues, and systemic imbalances, highlighting their wide range of applications.

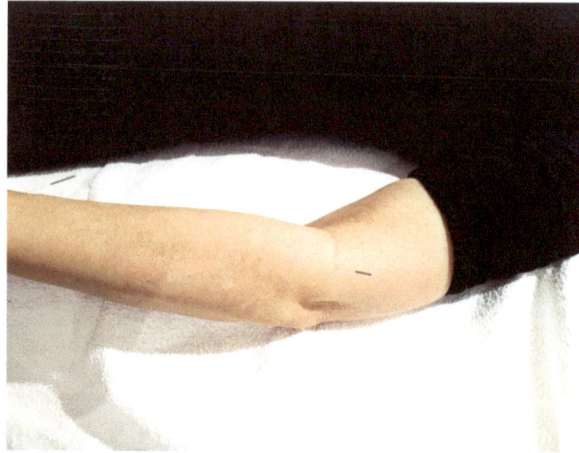

**Picture 29. It displays a needle is inserted at point LI11,
located on the large intestine energy channel.**

Your gastrointestinal tract, which is comparable in size to a large studio apartment, plays a significant role in the digestion of food, the absorption of nutrients, and, importantly, the regulation of water intake. Its substantial surface area is a key factor in these vital functions, ensuring your body maintains the right balance of fluids. Your skin weighs approximately kilograms and has a surface area of about 2 square meters. Skin is the body's largest organ. Women's skin is different, with a greater density of nerve sensors that increases sensitivity to touch, and pain compared to men.

If you are a woman, your feminine skin is smooth and soft, with elasticity and a more youthful appearance. In contrast, men's skin is thicker and more robust due to the presence of a greater number of collagen fibers.

Your gut releases over 20 hormones that regulate your metabolism, immune responses, and act as vital messengers between the gut, brain, and heart. Specifically, Ghrelin, a gut hormone, plays a crucial role in protecting your heart. It has significant cardio-protective effects, including reducing cardiac muscle thickness, if it is overgrown and its inflammation.

Ghrelin also accelerates programmed cell death known as apoptosis. It is a fundamental natural process. Millions of your corrupted cells agree daily to suicide for the sake of the integrity of your whole body, protecting you from cancer development from the cells that have already corrupted DNA.

The insertion of needles 19 and 20 accomplished the second stage of the 30 Needles Constellation Acupuncture.

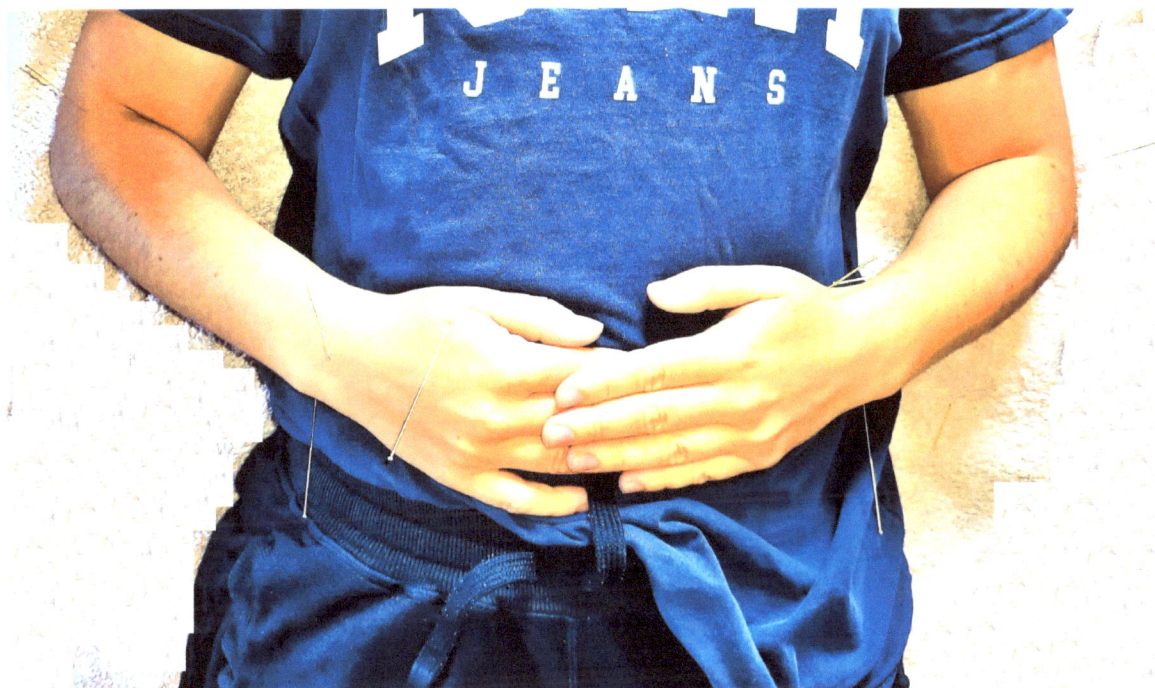

Picture 30. It displays all 8 inserted acupuncture needles, accomplishing stage two of the 30 Needles Constellation Acupuncture.

8

The third stage of the acupuncture treatment

Every man who comes into the world carries within a general chart of his life, the details of which he fills in throughout his lifetime. The highways, and some byways, are already in the chart when he is born. These are traits he brings with him from previous incarnations. You are born with about 75% of your life predetermined by your past. You will make up the remaining 25%. Paramahansa Yogananda.

The needles 21 to 30 on your legs have a strong impact on your epigenetic messenger RNA (mRNA). The activation of these points with acupuncture needles also regulates the DNA responses and the action of the molecular motors, your friendly *kinases*.

The needles 21 and 22 of the 30 Needles Constellation Acupuncture are inserted bilaterally at the acupuncture points ST36 of the stomach energy channel. The stomach energy channel forms a functional unit with the spleen energy channel. It starts under the eye and ends between the first and the second toe. It has 45 gateway points.

Acupuncture point ST36, also known as Zusanli or "leg three mile", is a renowned acupuncture point that offers rejuvenation, longevity, and vitality. Its name is steeped in a fascinating Chinese legend, adding a great value to its importance.

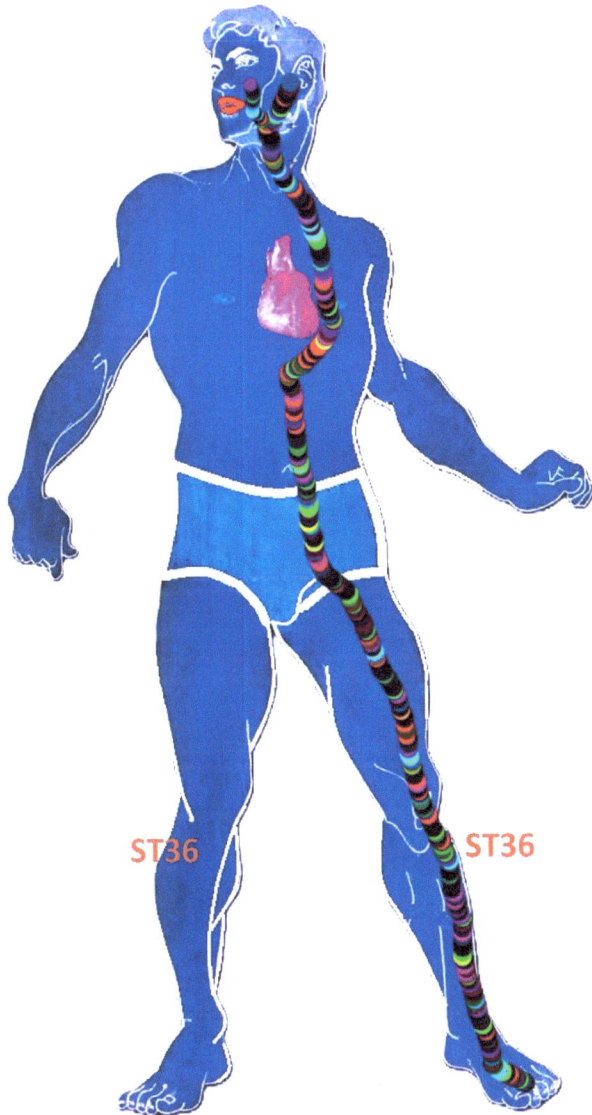

Picture 31. It displays the stomach energy channel. Acupuncture points ST36 are marked.

In Chinese, ST36 point is called Zusanli, which translates to "leg three mile". This name is rooted in a captivating legend from ancient times, when the only means of travel in China was on foot. Activating this point enabled one to walk an additional three miles, providing factual evidence of its revitalizing abilities for the body. The point ST36, a master point for all symptoms in the abdominal region. ST36 is a powerful entry point to calm any abdominal pains, such as indigestion, bloating, or cramps, as well as dysfunctions like constipation or diarrhea. It is used for local anesthesia with acupuncture needles inserted in the ST36 points during surgeries and to relieve pain during childbirth.

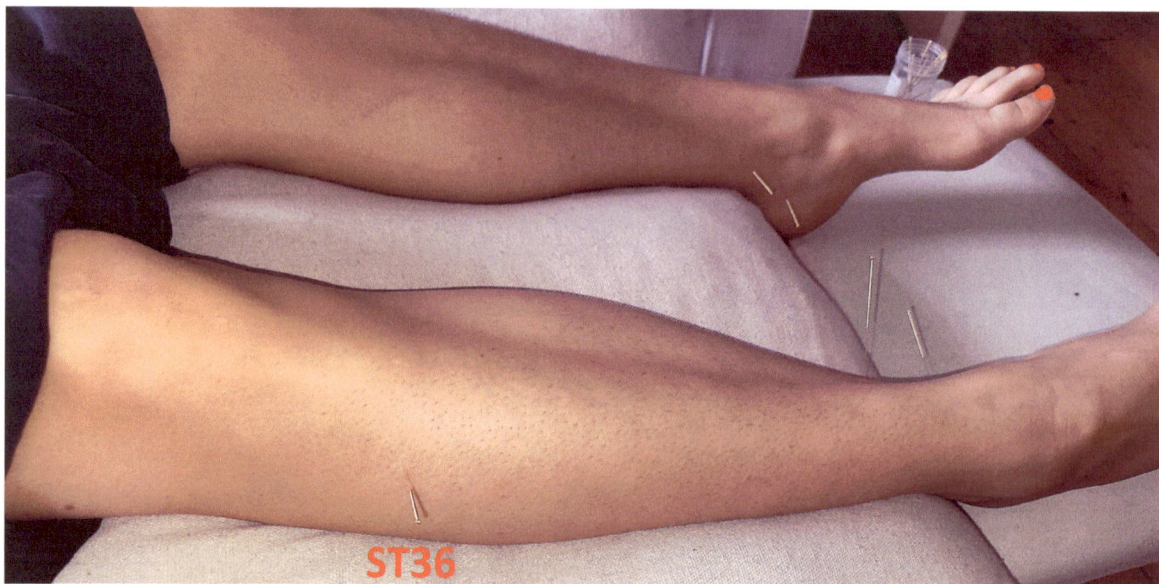

Picture 32. The image depicts an inserted needle at the acupuncture point ST36 of the stomach energy channel. Additionally, the needles at the points SP6 of the spleen energy channel above the ankle, and the K3 point of the kidney energy channel between the ankle bone and Achilles ligament are displayed.

The ST36 acupoints, when activated by acupuncture needles, facilitate the release of hormones and other signaling molecules, thereby positively affecting the stress response and the immune system. Studies show that ST36 stimulation releases hormones such as thyroid-stimulating hormone (TSH) and cortisol. It also activates the follicle-stimulating hormone (FSH), as well as neurotransmitters like endorphins and Ghrelin. These hormonal changes have wide-ranging systemic effects, mobilizing the energetic reserves of your body. These important hormones boost the anti-inflammatory defense and normalize your responses to pain. They play a role in reducing stress and invigorating your immune competent cells. The follicle-stimulating hormone (FSH) is vital for both men and women. It plays a crucial role in regulating libido, reproductive health, fertility, and overall hormonal balance in both men and women.

The needles 23 and 24 will be inserted at the acupuncture points GB34 Yuanglinquan of the gall bladder energy channel.

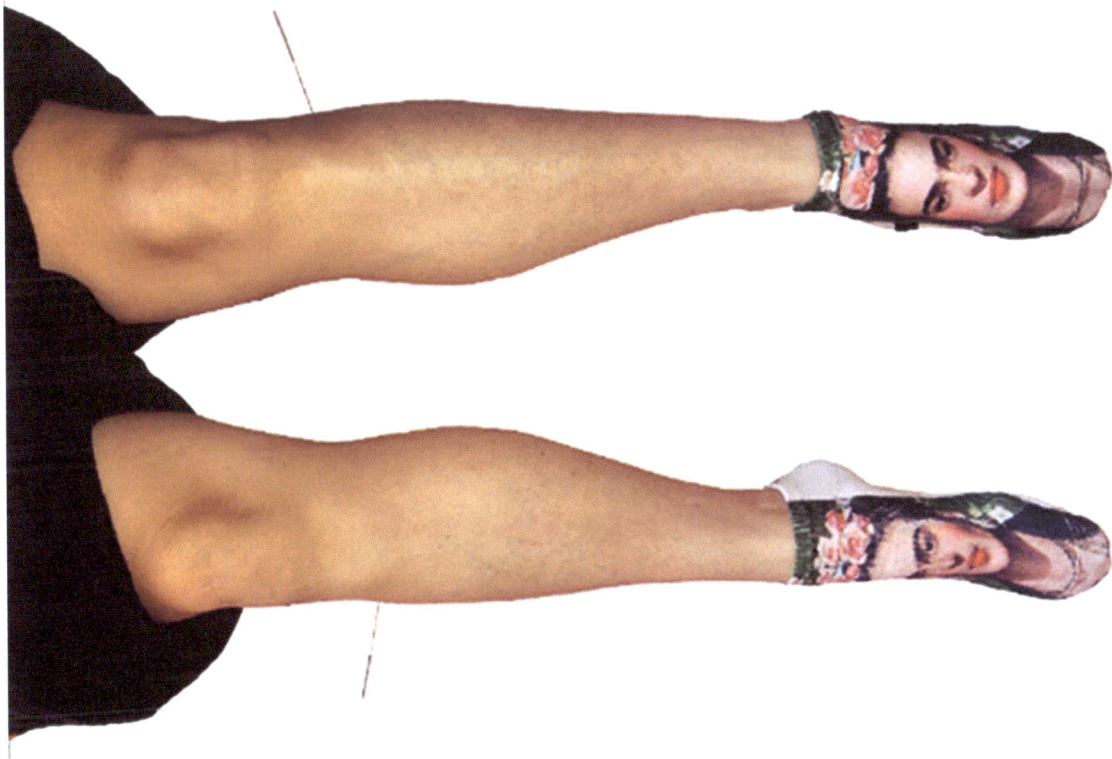

The stimulation of these points with acupuncture needles improves skin health and relaxes all tendons and ligaments in your body. It strengthens your adrenal glands and gives positive impulses to your genetics. The changes in your epigenetics refer not only to the potential of acupuncture to influence DNA, mRNA, and gene expression but also include improvement of your body's appearance.

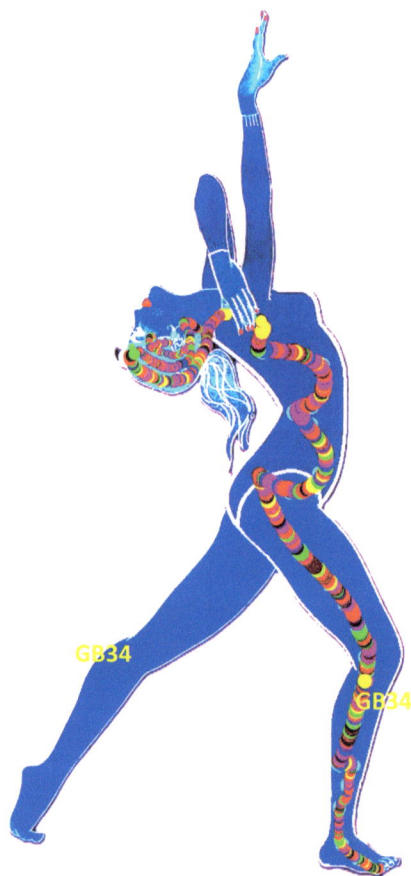

Picture 34. It displays the gallbladder energy channel.
The acupuncture points GB34 is marked.

The gall bladder energy channel starts at the head close to the eye, about 2 cm from its outside corner, and ends at the small toe of your foot. It has 44 gateway points.

Needles 25 and 26 are inserted at the acupuncture points K3 Taixi on the kidney energy channel.

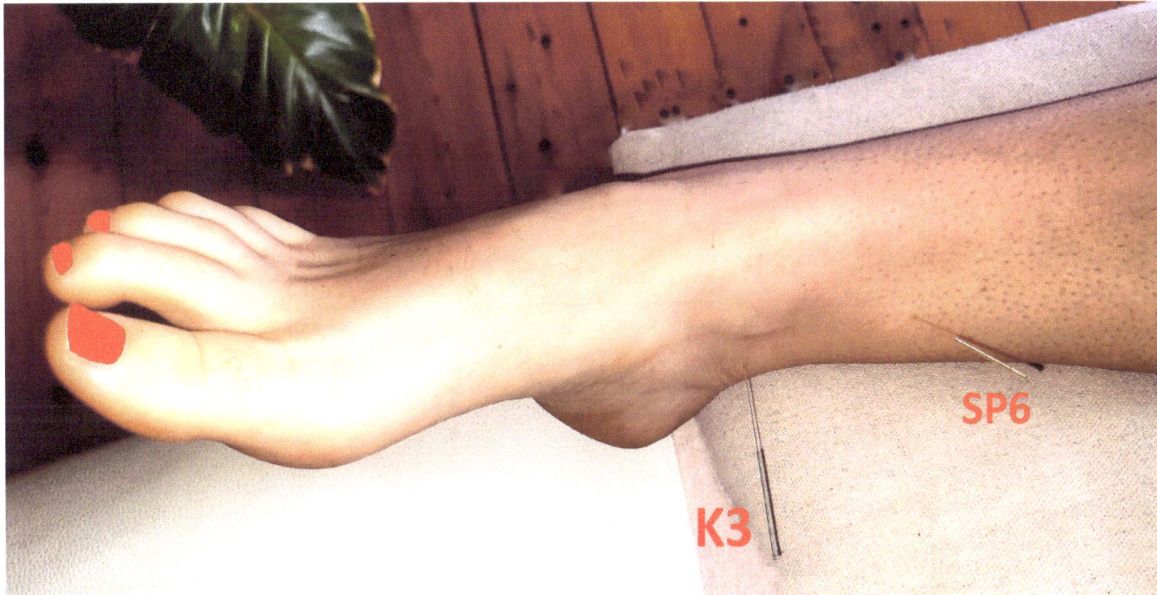

Picture 35. It displays the needles inserted at the acupuncture points K3 and SP6.

The needles 25 and 26 are inserted in the acupuncture point K3, also known as Taixi. The acupuncture point Taixi is located on the inside of the ankle, in the depression between the inner ankle bone and the Achilles tendon. It is a vital point on the kidney energy channel. Activation of this point with an acupuncture needle strengthens the kidney organ, improves sleep, balances the vital energy, and addresses symptoms such as fatigue, anxiety, and urinary leakage. The acupuncture point K3 can influence adrenal function via the brain-pituitary-adrenal axis. The brain-pituitary-adrenal axis is the body's primary stress response system. This complex hormonal network links the brain to the adrenal glands to regulate physiological and behavioral responses to internal and external stressors and maintains fluid balance.

The stimulating effect of adrenaline can be reduced, and the excitation or influence of other stress hormones can be calmed. Activation of the acupuncture point K3 with an acupuncture needle improves sleep and relieves pain.

Points SP6 and K3 form a powerful duo in the 30-Needles Constellation of Acupuncture. They are really hormonal points, and their activation releases feminine hormones and balances estrogen with progesterone. These two major hormones provide protection to the woman's heart and cardiovascular system.

The kidney energy channel originates in the middle of the forefoot, at the sole, and enters the interior of your body under the collarbone. It has 27 gateway points. It gives internal branches to the end of the spine, the kidneys, the heart, and the root of the tongue. You can use the entry points for your awareness training or reflexology.

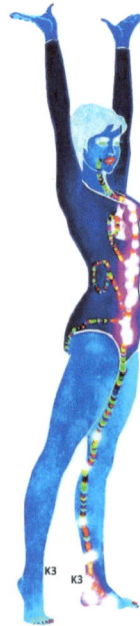

Picture 36. It displays the kidney energy channel. The acupuncture points K3 are marked.

The needles 27 and 28 of the 30 Needles Constellation Acupuncture are inserted bilaterally at point SP6 of the spleen energy channel. The spleen energy channel starts at the tip of the big toe, runs upwards inside the leg and thigh to the pelvic region close to the reproductive organs, and then goes up on the belly to the side of the cheek, at the height of the nipple, where it ends. It has two internal branches. One branch goes to the tongue and lips, and the other to the heart. The spleen channel has 21 gateway points.

The sixth point of the spleen energy channel SP 6 is a meeting point of the three Yin and the unification of the three feminine Yin energy channels. The spleen is located on the left-hand side of our body, between the stomach and the diaphragm. The spleen also has a function to filter, clean, and order our blood production. Red blood cells have a lifespan of around 120 days, after which your spleen breaks them down. In this process, old blood is destroyed by separating the old red blood cells, which are then recycled for their vital components like iron. The spleen also acts as a filter for our blood, cleansing it from bacteria, viruses, and other protein debris. It is essential to fight effectively against all starting infections. When blood flows through your spleen, white blood cells attack and remove any foreign invaders. Before birth, in the uterus, the baby produces red and white blood cells in the spleen. Shortly before birth, the spleen loses its ability to produce red blood cells, and the bone marrow takes over this function.

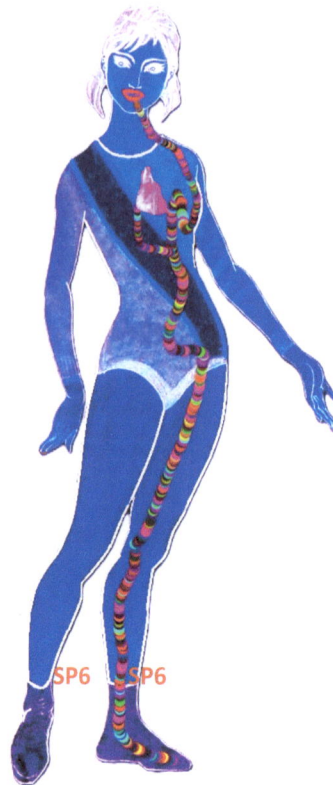

**Picture 37. It displays the spleen energy channel. The
acupuncture points SP6 are marked.**

The needle inserted at the point SP6 activates the release of Oxytocin, the hormone of your pi-tuitary gland located in the brain. It modulates the intensity of sexual encounters and impacts the movements of the uterus. It is crucial for childbirth that Oxytocin stimulates uterine contractions to induce labor.   Thereby, it should be exercised extreme caution when using needles or stimulat-ing this point through reflexology before 37 weeks pregnancy. In practice, therapists should consider this SP6 point in the same manner as other sensitive acupuncture points, such as LI4 on the large intestine energy channel, with which you are already familiar.

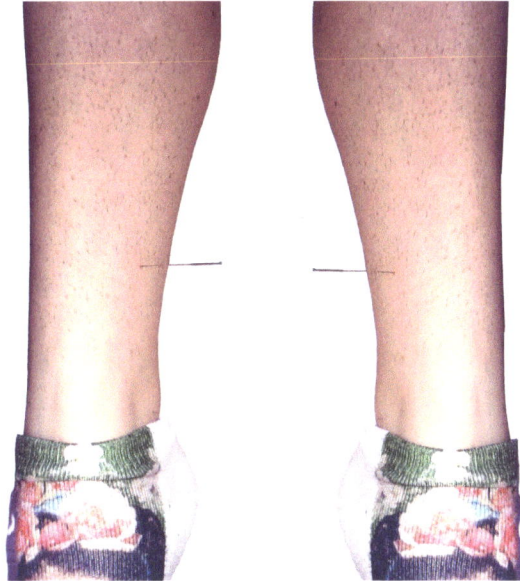

Picture 38. It displays acupuncture needles inserted in the points SP6.

The SP6 acupuncture point is the master or Command point related to hormonal imbalance. It stimulates the release and balance of estrogen and progesterone; therefore, its stimulation with the acupuncture needle should be considered in conditions such as irregular periods, PMS, or menopause symptoms. The SP6 of the spleen energy channels is the meeting point with the liver and kidney energy channels, all yin and feminine in their nature. Therefore, it is a significant point and it is used in acupuncture treatment for all women's infirmities. The spleen also determines the reactivity and the strength of your immune system. It also accelerates detox through the lymphatic system, particularly in the pelvic region.

According to traditional medicine, the spleen is considered the driving force behind the immune system. It dominates your blood and your digestive functions, as well as the production of nutrients vital for muscle activity. It transforms the nutrients digested in the stomach into protein for the muscles. It produces specific blood components, including immune-competent cells. It induces the immune response to any infection, ensuring your body's defense mechanisms are always guarding you. You can use the spleen energy channel entry points for self-reflexology or bodily awareness training.

The popular saying for the spleen function and its diagnostics in Chinese medicine is: "spleen looks through the lips". It has diagnostic meaning in case of herpes virus eruptions on the lips. Almost all of us are carriers of this type of virus as an attachment to our DNA. So, nearly everyone has, from time to time, cold sores, which are fluid-filled blisters that typically form on or near the lips. It manifests only when your immune system becomes weak.

The needles 29 and 30 are two needles placed bilaterally at the point LIV3 of the liver energy channel. The liver energy channel originates between the 1st and 2nd toes and ascends the front of the body toward the belly. It makes a loop to the reproductive organs and then reaches the liver on the right side of the abdomen. The liver energy channel has 14 gateway points. Then, the liver channels internal branches inside the body to the voice box region and curves around the lips. Going further upwards connects to the eyes and brain. LIV3 acupuncture point, also known as Taichong, translates from Chinese to "Great Surge of Energy." Inserting the needles in these acupuncture points not only energizes the liver energy channel but also has a profound calming effect, satisfying the body's need for energy.

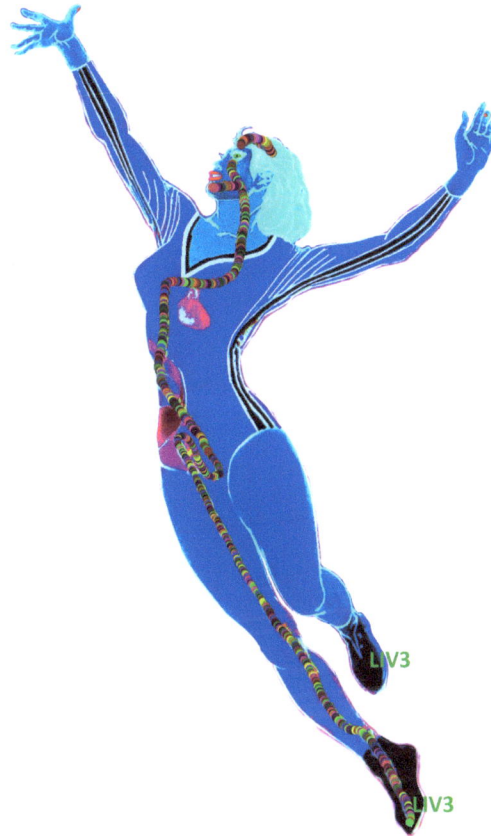

Picture 39. It displays the liver energy channel. The acupuncture points LIV3 are marked.

This point is used to regulate the flow of vital energy, calm the mind, and soothe stress and anger. It can also help with issues such as low back pain, high blood pressure, and insomnia. The 30 Needles Constellation Acupuncture ultimately lets you feel relaxed and at ease, as you have left the special recharge room for your body and soul, and not merely the treatment table.

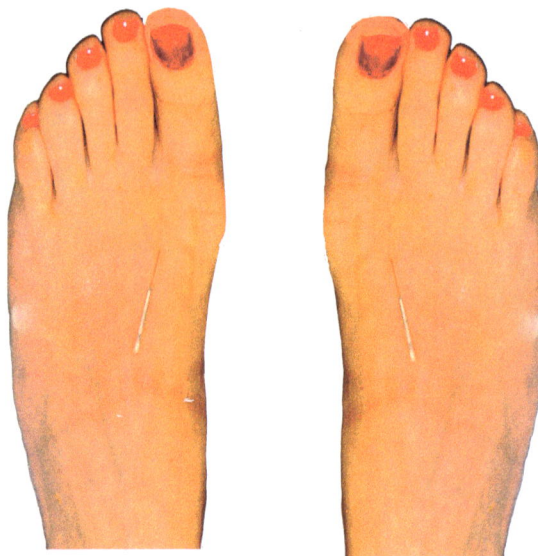

Picture 40. The needles are inserted at points LIV3 of the liver energy channel.

The acupuncture point LIV3 is associated with hormone regulation and stress reduction. It stimulates the adrenal glands and supports the body's natural hormonal balance. The activation of the acupuncture LIV3 points will restore your balance, ease menstrual discomfort, and reduce anxiety, which can indirectly impact hormonal processes. Traditionally, the primary functions of the LIV3 point include calming the liver fire, regulating blood flow, improving vision, and stimulating lymphatic flow. Research indicates that acupuncture at this point accelerates the lymphatic flow, with some studies showing improvements in symptoms of lymphatic swelling.

9

The Centre. The needle GV26 unlocks your breathing

Jesus said to them again, "Peace be with you. As the Father has sent me, even so I am sending you". Then he breathed on them and said, "Receive the Holy Spirit". John Chapter 20, Verse 22-23.

The point GV26, Shuigou, after translation into English, is "The Centre". The acupuncture point is GV26 located above the upper lip. It belongs to the brain meridian, which runs from the crotch alongside your entire spine on your back. It further ascends through the middle of your head, then runs down from the top of your head to the upper lip. The front part of the brain meridian travels over the mid-line of your body between the bottom lip and the crotch. Your mouth, lips, and tongue form a link and unite the brain energy channel. The acupuncture point GV26 is the meeting point of feminine yin and masculine yang energy. It is "The Centre" between these two opposite elements. Therefore, activation of this point with an acupuncture needle can effectively reinforce the joint energy of yin and yang, even bringing a person back to full awareness after a fainting incident. The Shuigou acupuncture point, GV26, is often impacted by injuries, traumas such as car accidents or falls, or prolonged stress load on your heart due to work pressure or personal crises. It leads to blockages or stagnation in the circular flow of your breathing energy.

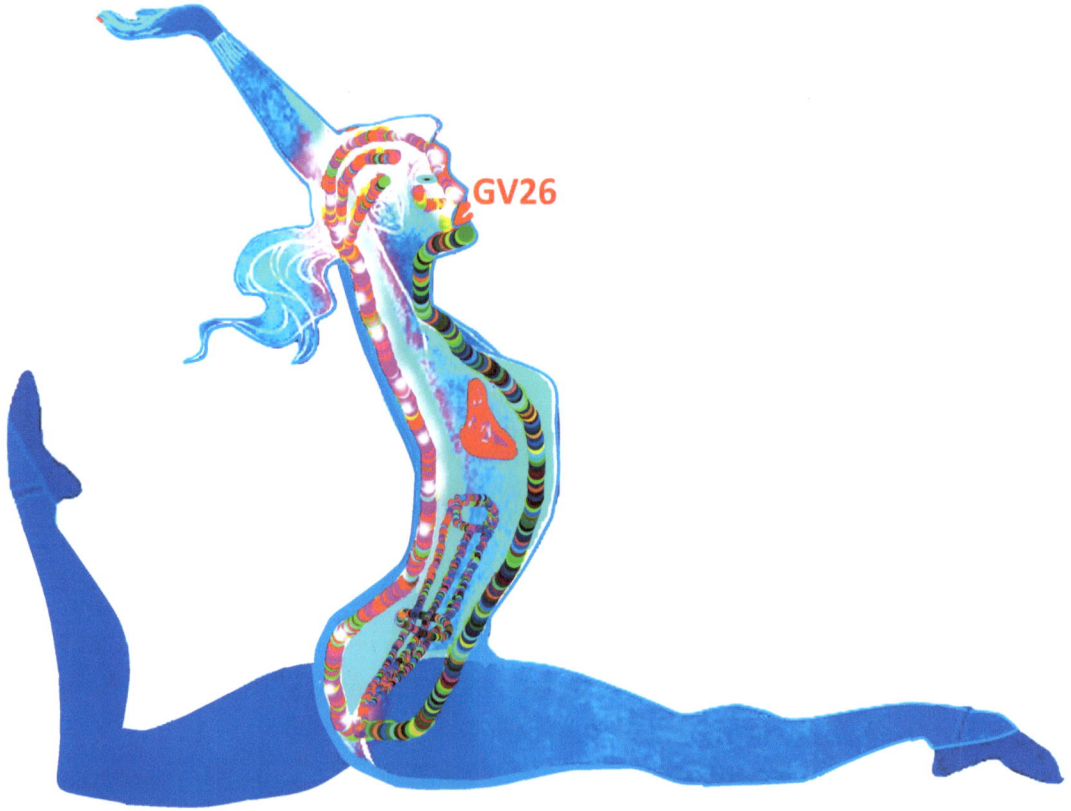

Picture 41. It displays the GV26 point, "The Centre" of the brain meridian.

It is a poignant reminder of how your body responds to stress, both physical and psychological, by creating muscle armoring, a constriction of muscles in a reflex to protect your internal organs. Your body's chronic state of tension and rigidity, often resulting from trauma or prolonged stress, can be released by treating this very special point with acupuncture.

It is beneficial to remember that in situations where a person is about to pass out or is experiencing lightheadedness or dizziness, stimulation of GV26 with the acupuncture needle can prompt or correct the vital breathing flow of energy, and can help restore spontaneous, deep breathing after a fainting episode.

In the treatment of fainting, the insertion of the acupuncture needle on the GV26 point may quickly increase blood pressure and stimulate respiration in a person who has experienced a fainting episode. The acupuncture point GV26 is also commonly used for acute neurological conditions, acute low back strain, and sciatica. The acupuncture point GV26, located above your upper lip, is a very special acupuncture point, as it is essential for the smooth flow of your orbital breathing.

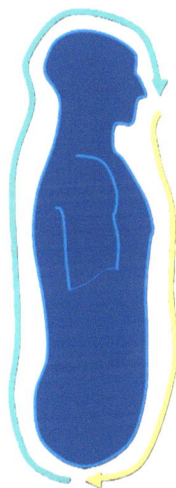

Picture 42. It displays the Microcosmic orbit by Bostjan46. Own work, CC0, https://commons. Wikimedia.

The brain energy channel and its partner, the spinal cord, are intertwined with your breathing. This is a profound revelation and the solid evidence of the holistic nature of your body. Practicing orbital breathing will increase the oxygenation of all internal organs and invigorate your brain. This is a safe way to maintain your health and boost your vitality.

The brain meridian, a key component of the 14 energy channels, is a fascinating area of study. Your brain meridian has 51 acupuncture entry points, and it is not accidental that its route coincides with the energy flow alongside the orbit for breathing. Better understanding the brain meridian can unlock a wealth of knowledge about your body's energy flow.

You have the power to consciously speed up the vital energy flow into your brain with each deep breath and awareness of the path, as your breath energy orbits. This conscious control enables you to achieve your perfect health and radiant well-being.

The inhalation energy flows from the crotch, travels along your entire spine, and reaches the middle of your head, ending at the area between the nose and the upper lip, at the acupuncture point "The Centre".

As you focus on the circular energy flow, you are fully present and aware of yourself practicing the advanced art of breathing, which boosts the vital energy flow to your brain. The GV26, situated above your upper lip, is a key acupuncture point for unlocking your breathing. This point is often affected by significant stress, both physical and psychological.

There have been emergency situations in your life. When high stress impacts your body as it occurs due to traumas, a car accident, or facing violence, you involuntarily create 'muscle armor'. This neuro-muscular reflex causes the blockage of vital energy at the GV26 acupuncture point. Muscle armoring is a quick reflex that tightens essential muscles deep within your body to protect your internal organs. This reflex, which occurs in seconds, also disrupts the natural rhythm and flow of breathing, causing a blockage of vital energy at the GV26 acupuncture point. In this moment of trauma, you also stopped the natural rhythm and flow of breathing.

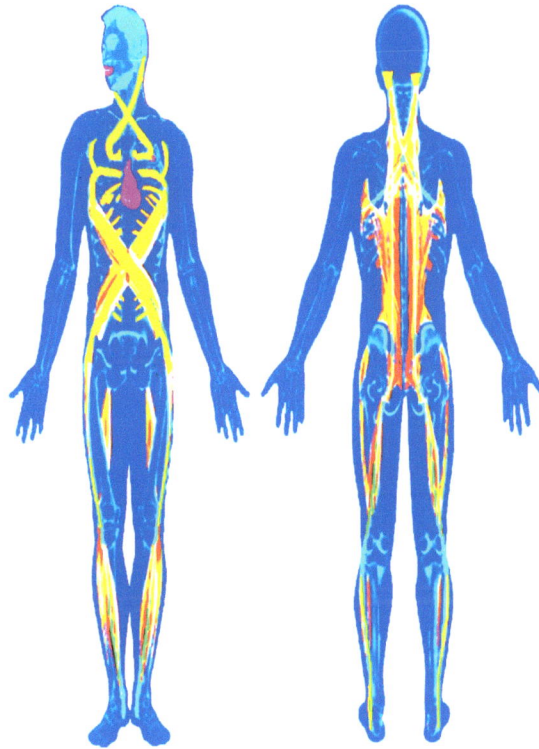

Picture 43. It depicts the muscle armoring.

"Muscle armor" is a somatic indicator of how stress, both physical and psychological, triggers your body's defense mechanism, resulting in muscle constriction to protect vital organs. Still, it disrupts your natural breathing rhythm.

The needles placed at the last point of the large intestine energy channel, Li 20 -Yingxiang, support the free flow of your breath. The Chinese name Yingxiang, which means "Welcome fragrances", adds a unique cultural dimension to the functionality of this acupuncture point. The needles at the points LI20 on both sides of the nose facilitate effective breathing and improve the ability to distinguish between fragrances and odors. LI20 is an acupuncture point in the energy channel of the Large Intestine. Yingxiang is the main point for the good functioning of your nose and for sensing a variety of fragrances.

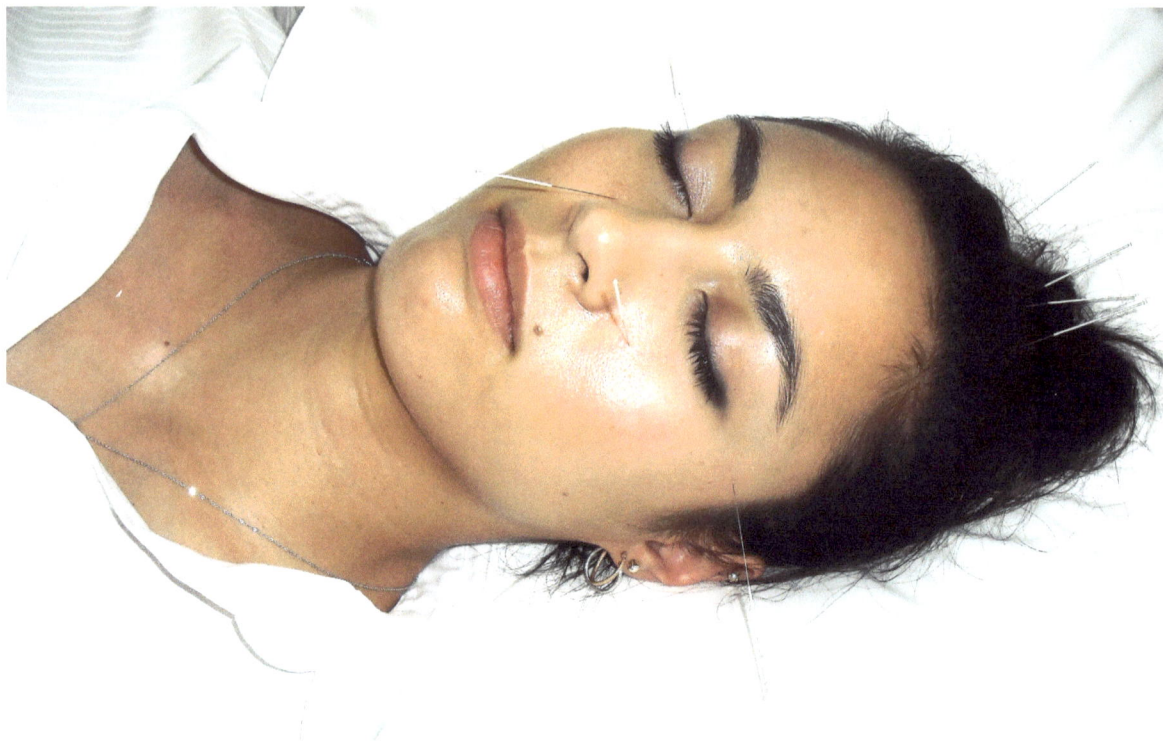

Picture 44. It displays the acupuncture needles at the points LI20 of the large intestine energy channel, on the cheeks, beside the nose. The needles are also inserted in the extra-point ShiShenCong at the top of the head and in the extra-point Taiyang at the temples.

The pathway a scent begins when airborne molecules enter the nasal cavity. This thin tissue, located high in the nasal cavity, contains millions of sensors for smell. Each of these sensors is designed to bind with specific fragrance molecules. Stimulation with the acupuncture needles at points LI20 supports the GV26 acupuncture point in the unlocking of your breathing mechanism, thereby enhancing the oxygenation of your body and brain. This stimulation not only improves your breathing but also replenishes your life energy, giving you more control over your energy resources. You can feel more alert and energetic after acupuncture at LI20. You may experience improved digestion or better sleep. These are all examples of how LI20 activation can replenish your life energy. The large intestine energy channel starts with the index finger and ends at the cheek beside the nose on the opposite side. It has 20 gateway points.

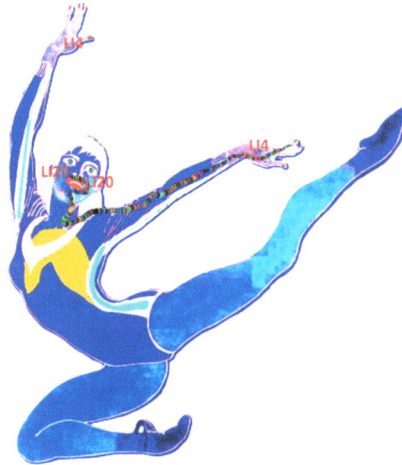

**Picture 45. It displays the large intestine energy channel.
The acupuncture points LI20 and LI4 are marked.**

10

30 Needles Constellation Acupuncture Plus

Absolute, unquestioning faith in God is the greatest method of instantaneous healing. Paramahansa Yogananda.

In the following years of my acupuncture practice, I observed that some patients had specific symptoms, such as Tinnitus, insomnia, inflammation of the pericardium (the sac surrounding the heart), or lower back pain. These conditions often require a few more needles.

Building on this observation, I have incorporated the **30 Needles Constellation Acupuncture Plus** into my practice. The additional acupuncture points I have selected for these conditions included **PC6**, an acupuncture point of the pericardium energy channel, **SI3**, a point of the small intestine energy channel, **Yintang**, an extra acupuncture point located between the eyebrows, which targets the 'Third Eye', and **GB20**, a point of the gallbladder energy channel. The point **ST4** of the stomach energy channel is also sometimes included in the **30 Needles Constellation Acupuncture Plus.**

The expansion of the number of needles improved the effectiveness of my acupuncture treatments. The higher number of needles I have been using in treating Tinnitus and its associated symptoms, such as vertigo, dizziness, extreme sound sensitivity, ear pain or fullness, pulsating sounds that match the heartbeat, and even jaw pain. Depending on the underlying cause, Tinnitus can also lead to significant psychological effects like anxiety, depression, stress, and sleep problems. The constant noise can interfere with your ability to focus and your concentration.

The PC6 is the sixth entry point of the pericardium energy channel. This acupuncture point is also known as Neiguan. It means in English " The Inner Gate". It is located on the inner forearm, 4cm above the wrist crease, between the two large tendons.

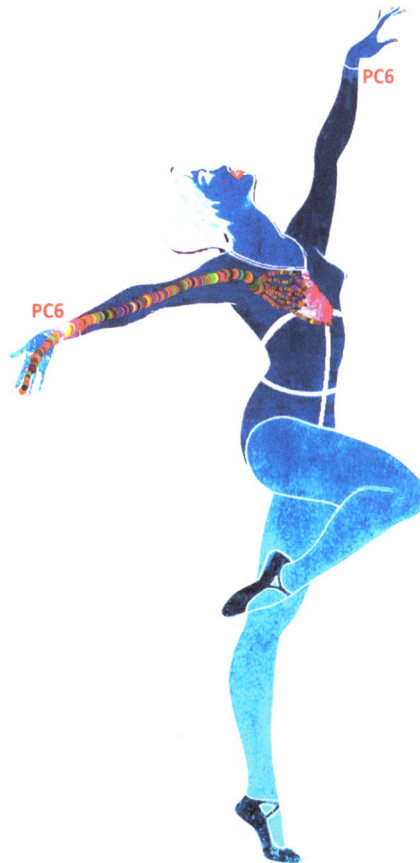

**Picture. 46. It displays the pericardium energy channel.
The acupuncture points PC6 are marked.**

Stimulating Neiguan with an acupuncture needle can significantly boost your immunity, which is closely connected to the lymphatic system. The pericardium, acting as the motor for lymph movement, serves as the body's first line of defense. It's like a molecular sieve, where bacteria and viruses are trapped and eliminated by immune-competent cells, providing a solid foundation for your body's defense system.

The acupuncture at **the PC6** point also influences the complex pattern in the brain. It is therefore used to treat nausea, vomiting, and motion sickness, and also anxiety and pain relief. Research confirms that PC6 stimulation helps improve symptoms of hypertension and Angina pectoris, the chest pain caused by spasms of the coronary arteries. Activation of the PC6 with an acupuncture needle benefits the weakened heart muscle.

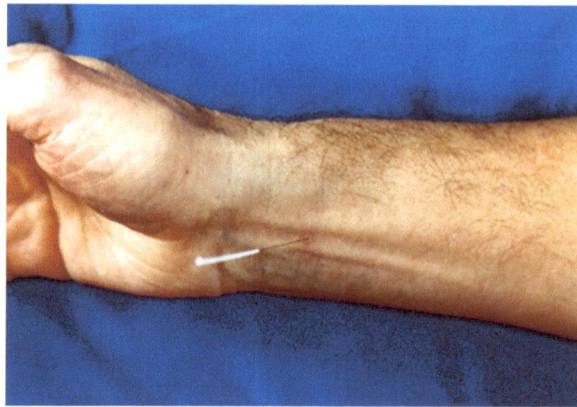

Picture 47. It displays the needle at the acupuncture point PC6 of the pericardium energy channel.

Stimulating **PC6** triggers the release of specific neurotransmitters, such as GABA and serotonin, which are known to enhance mood. This can leave you feeling uplifted and positive, contributing to your overall well-being. According to traditional practice, PC6 plays a crucial role in harmonizing the stomach and small intestine, which are related to various digestive maladies caused by emotional issues, thereby connecting you to their emotional roots.

Another additional point, included in the **30 Needles Constellation Plus**, is the **SI3** acupuncture point of the small intestine energy channel, also known as Houxi, which translates to "Back Ravine" in English.

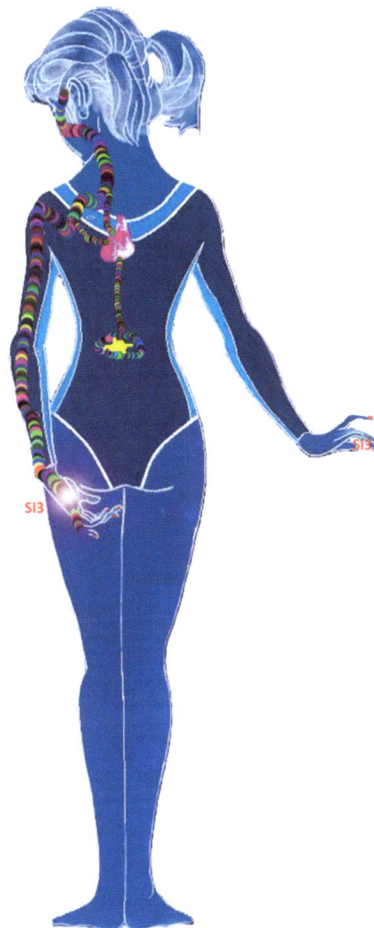

**Picture 48. It displays the small intestine energy channel.
Acupuncture points SI3 are marked.**

This translation vividly describes the action of the acupuncture needle, which can turn your lower back from a condition where your spinal disc is trapped between the bones of your spine. This situation is a ravine situation where your spinal nerves are between "the rock" of your vertebra and a spinal disc, another hard place. The small intestine energy channel starts at your small finger and ends just below the eye. It has 19 gateway points. It has two branches that supply the heart: the solar plexus and the small intestine. The entry point SI3 is an acupuncture point located on the outer side of your hand, in a depression just above the head of the fifth smallest finger. Activating the SI3 acupuncture point with a needle is a proven method for treating tensions in your neck or lower back pain.

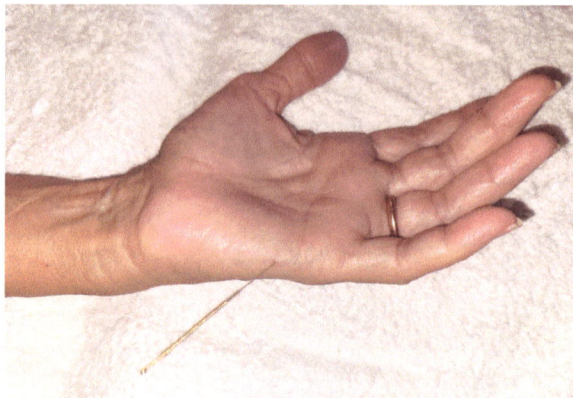

Picture 49. It displays a needle inserted at the acupuncture point SI3 of the small intestine energy channel.

The following fascinating acupuncture point, which I added to the **30 Needles Constellation Acupuncture Plus**, is an extra point **called Yintang**. Yintang is an extra single acupuncture point. The location of the Yintang acupuncture point is also known as the 'Third Eye'. It is situated between the eyebrows. It is located in front of your ethmoid bone. The ethmoid bone, with its unique spongy and perforated structure, is exceptional in its nature. It is equipped with electromagnetic sensors. Your profound connection with this entry point can inspire you to explore the depths of your own intuition and inner vision as part of the electromagnetic sensing process.

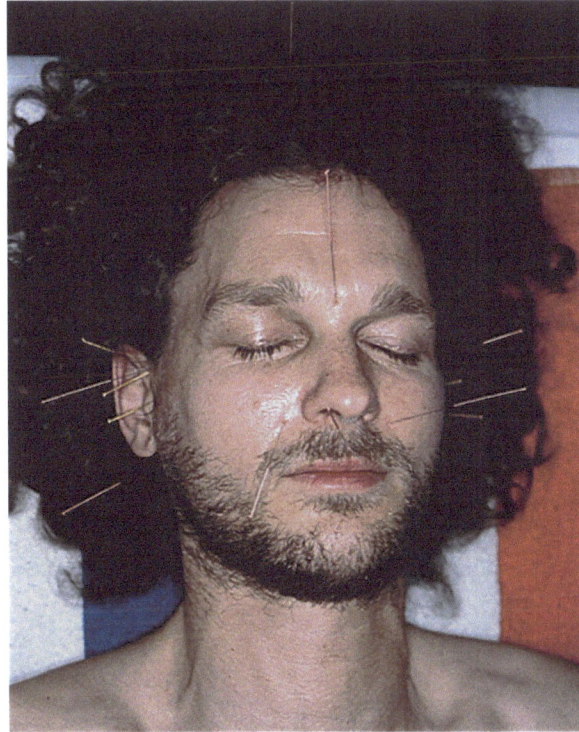

Picture 50. It displays the first stage of the 30-Needles Constellation Acupuncture Plus, including the head and face. A single needle is inserted at the extra acupuncture point Yintang, located between the eyebrows, known as the "Third Eye". Additionally, several needles are inserted around each ear, forming the "Gate to the Ear" for Tinnitus treatment.

The name Yintang means in English the "Hall of Impressions" or "Hall of Scal", is an extra-acupuncture point. In the spiritual context of traditional medicine, it is often referred to as the "Third Eye", a place deeply associated with insight and inner vision in both Eastern and Western cultures. The needle inserted at the Yintang acupuncture point brings calmness and tranquility, much like the gentle touch of moonlight can make you peaceful and aware of your body and your entire environment, enhancing your sense of well-being.

I have found that acupuncture is not just a potential, but an effective treatment for Tinnitus. More than 50% of my patients were healed from Tinnitus, as shown in a study performed by my team and me. The acupuncture treatment for Tinnitus included inserting three needles into specific points, **SI19**, Tinggong in translation to English "Palace of Hearing", **SJ21**, Ermen in translation to English "Ear Gate", both of the small intestine energy channel, and **GB2,** Tinghui in translation to English "Meeting of Hearing", of the gall bladder energy channel. These three entry points build the "Gate to the Ear" area. Depending on the underlying cause, with this extended number of needles, Tinnitus-related significant psychological effects like anxiety, depression, stress, and sleep problems were improved.

The acupuncture point **GB20**, Fengchi, is a key element in the **30 Needles Constellation Acupuncture Plus.** Also known as "The Wind Pool", it is a pivotal meeting point for several key energy channels, including the gallbladder, triple energizer, and other internal energy channels. Located at the base of the skull, it plays a crucial role in acupuncture, particularly in the removal of external influences or internal wind caused by emotions. Activation of this points with an acupuncture needles also improves headaches, neck pain, and flu symptoms. It is also an important acupuncture point in the treatment of Tinnitus.

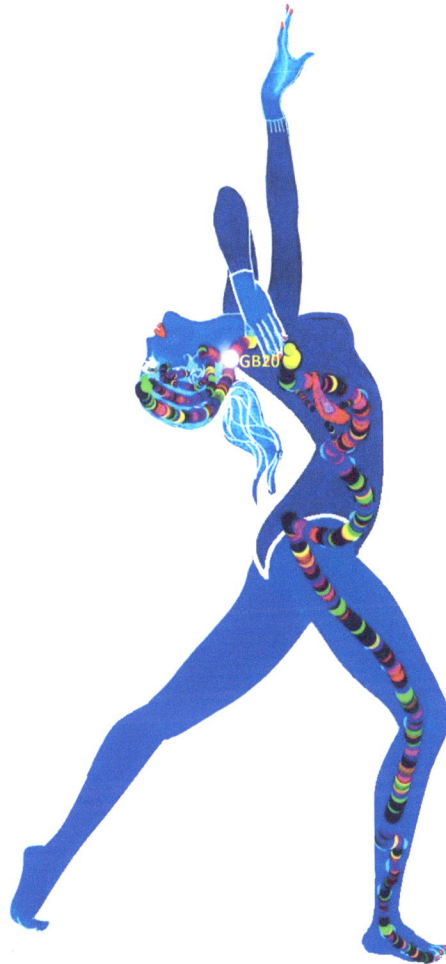

**Picture 51. It displays the gallbladder energy channel.
The acupuncture point GB20 is marked.**

The acupuncture point ST4 of the stomach energy channel is another acupuncture point included in the **30 Needles Constellation Acupuncture Plus**. It is known as Dicang. It translates into English as 'The Earth Granary'. It is located laterally to the corner of the mouth. It is a 'meeting point', a term in acupuncture that signifies a point where two or more energy channels intersect, in this case, for the stomach and large intestine energy channels.

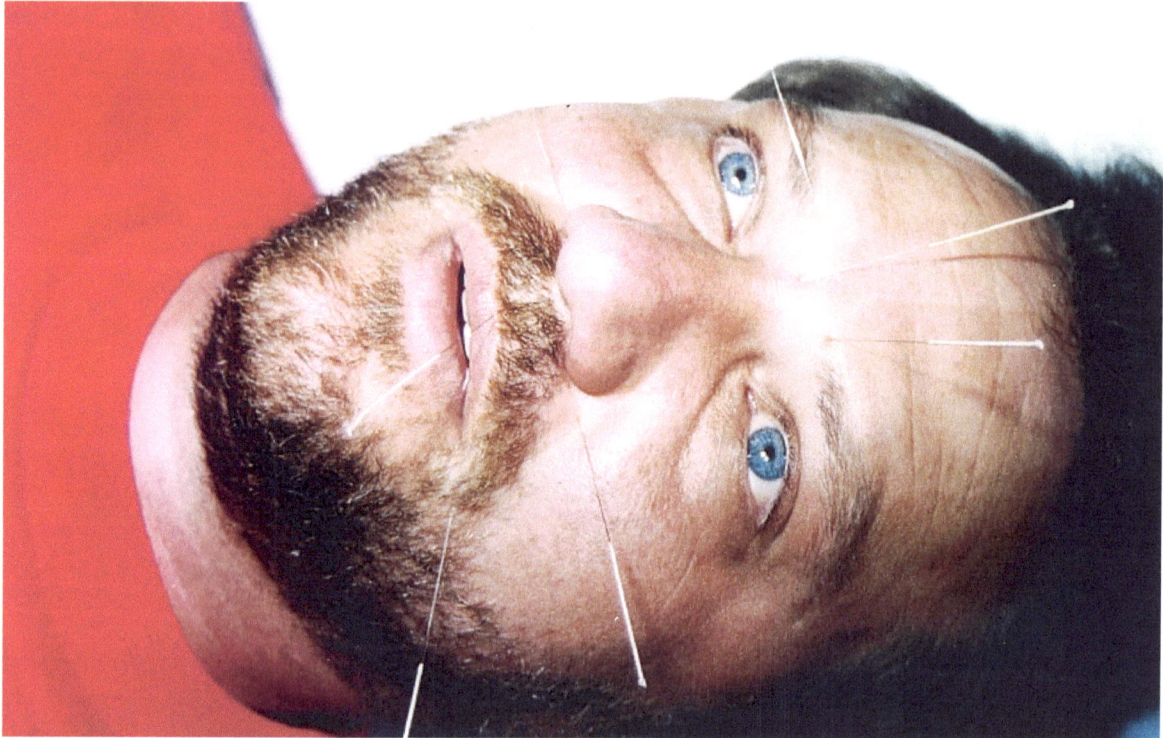

Picture 52. It displays a needle inserted into the acupuncture point ST4, located at the corner of the mouth of the stomach energy channel.

Its name, 'The Earth Granary', refers to its connection to the nourishing elements related to the spleen and stomach energy channel. Acupuncture point ST4 of the stomach energy channel is also used to treat facial pain and paralysis, eye twitching, and mouth deviations, while also acting as a "grounding" point to calm the face. Activation of the ST4 points corrects muscles that lift the face and relaxes those that pull it down. Therefore, the activation of the ST4 points also can help to reduce sagging in the lower face and changing the appearance of unhappiness.

The **30 Needles Constellation Acupuncture Plus** is designed to treat specific symptoms and special conditions, such as Tinnitus, with a thorough and comprehensive approach. This extended acupuncture treatment usually requires four or more needles, even up to 10 additional and necessary needles. The treatment of Tinnitus, a condition characterized by a ringing or buzzing in the ears, involves the total number of the inserted needles, which can be 40 or more, ensuring comprehensive and effective treatment that leaves no aspect of your condition overlooked. The 30-Needles Constellation Acupuncture offers you hope for significant improvement in your condition and symptoms and more often even healing.

It is important to note that the number of acupuncture needles used in this book is only an estimate. Your acupuncturist or doctor will tailor the treatment to your specific condition and the severity of the illness, ensuring you receive the most effective and personalized care.

11

Acupuncture changes your bodily appeal

The moment you change your perception is the moment you rewrite the chemistry of your body. Dr Bruce Lipton.

The modern life with a high load of stress and the environmental factors like UV radiation, pollution, diet, and lack of sleep can trigger epigenetic changes by turning genes "on" or "off", leading to visible signs of skin aging, such as wrinkles, hyper-pigmentation, reduced elasticity, and poor skin tone.

The 30 Needles Constellation Acupuncture and the **30 Needles Constellation Acupuncture Plus** approach play a significant role in controlling gene expression related to your stress load, intellectual power, and skin health. By regularly experiencing acupuncture treatment as a preventive measure and adopting a new lifestyle, you will notice changes in your overall appearance, primarily in rejuvenation. You may discover something new, the grace in your movements.

By changing the epigenetics, acupuncture can positively influence your character and personality expression. It allows your body, as a self-organizing system, to bring your intellectual health potential to its fullness. Acupuncture deploys molecular motors, triggers chemical changes that result in epigenetic marks, which control which genes are turned on or off. Acupuncture treatment regularly has a powerful influence on normal cell development, cell differentiation, maintaining cell identity, and cellular memory, empowering you to shape your own personality.

Acupuncture is not just about your body health and your well-being. It also affects your brain development, leading to notable positive variations in behavior, awareness, and personality. This intriguing aspect of acupuncture's influence on the heart, mind, soul, and body is evidence of its holistic impact on you. When the heart, mind, soul, and body work in harmony, it creates a graceful smoothness in your body movements, as well as an attractive, elegant appearance. It is the true meaning of the teaching *"The WHOLE is greater than the sum of its parts"*.

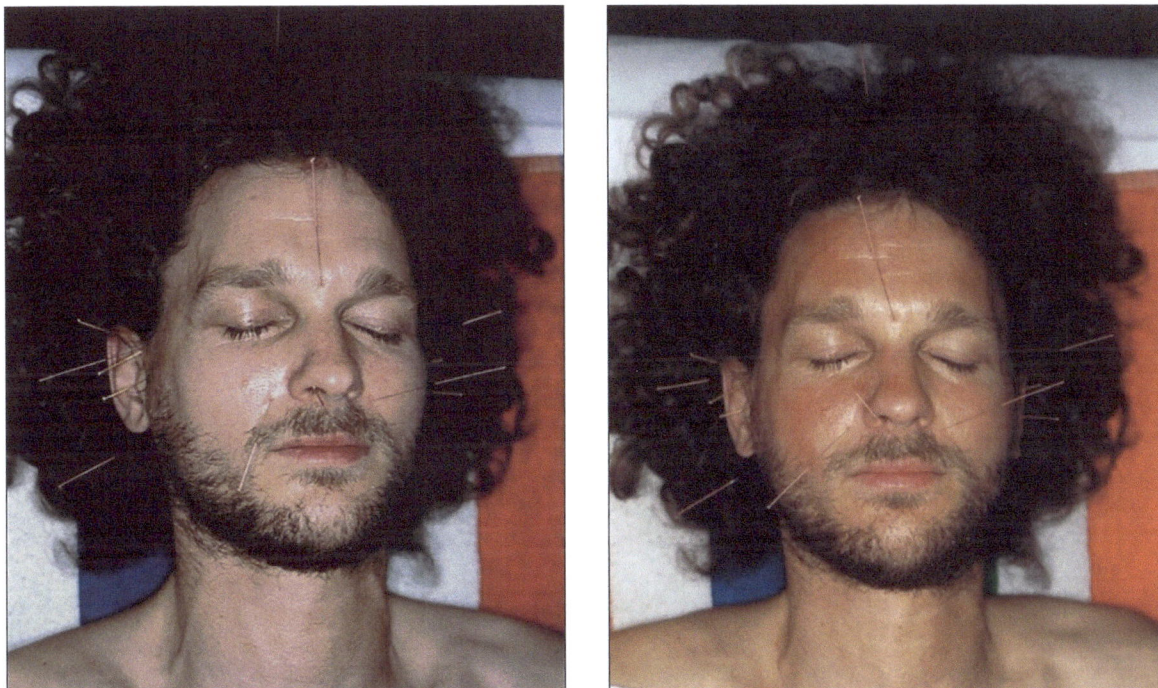

Picture 53. It displays a difference in the appearance of a same person before and after 30 Needles Constellation Acupuncture Plus.

This picture displays the same person at the beginning of the **30-Needle Constellation Acupuncture Plus** treatment on the left side and after 30 minutes of acupuncture treatment on the right side. Notably, after 30 minutes of acupuncture, the genuine 'body appeal' has changed. The skin appears to have improved blood supply; the shoulder line is relaxed, his face is broader, and his eyes are more comfortable. Please notice that even his hair is more toned and energized. More importantly, he is in a heightened state of awareness of his body. It appears that after acupuncture treatment, the mind and body are in real harmony.

Acupuncture has a positive influence on epigenetics, which can improve your appearance by affecting how genes are expressed, thereby establishing new epigenetic patterns. These new patterns are a bridge between your new experiences with acupuncture and the development of your new bodily characteristics. This can influence the facial expression and relaxation of the body, as well as the balance of muscles necessary for toning and other muscles that benefit from the relaxation patterns.

Acupuncture will improve your "bodily appeal," increasing your physical attractiveness and charm. The deeper awareness of your body after acupuncture treatment will be more radiant and attractive, and a striking aspect of your improved bodily expression will draw the attention of others.

Acupuncture can even improve the appearance of your hair by keeping it energized, toned, healthy, and strong.

Dear friend, I pray that you may enjoy good health and that all may go well with you, even as your soul is getting along well. 3 John Chapter 1, Verse 2.

Dr Jerzy George Dyczynski is a holistic cardiologist, Doctor of Medical Sciences, and a seasoned Acupuncturist with extensive international medical experience in both Western and Eastern countries. This profound international medical practice distinguishes him with a unique approach that combines conventional, modern, and holistic medicine. He has dedicated his career to empowering patients and promoting holistic, individualized health.

Dr. George is also an author, and his published works include "The Dyczynski Program. Healing the Intelligent Heart," published in 2022.

The newest series, "Medical Knowledge Made Easy," launched in 2024, is designed to simplify complex medical topics and make them accessible to everyone.

1.   Grace in Movement. The Training of Your Energy Channels for Better Health and Performance (2024).
2.   Positive Heart Remodeling. Heal Your Heart Adverse Remodeling (2024).
3.   Your Healing Hands. The Power of Reflexology (2024).
4.   Cardiology for Women. Your Heart in Distress (2025).
5.   30 Needles Constellation Acupuncture (2025).

These five books in this series can guide you in your quest to achieve perfect health; they make the modern heart stress load understandable. They provide awareness and physical training, along with a step-by-step description of how to benefit from your body as a self-organizing system. All books are written in a language that is understandable to everyone and highlight achievable health solutions.

Dr George's latest publication, "Cardiology for Women," published in early 2025, focuses specifically on holistic practices and women's unique heart health, empowering women to take control of their heart health.

This book, 30 Needles Constellation Acupuncture, focuses on holistic acupuncture. It is the fifth book in the "Medical Knowledge Made Easy" series and is a practical guide for everyone interested in whole-person healing through acupuncture.

In this acupuncture book, Dr. George shares with the world unique and practical knowledge acquired over more than 35 years of practice, the technique of practical and holistic acupuncture.

The 30 Needles Constellation Acupuncture is a treasure of ancient acupuncture wisdom. It is now revealed to enthusiasts of acupuncture and natural medicine, empowering you, the Reader, with tools for your healing journey and understanding the positive influence of acupuncture needles on your body's self-organizing system.

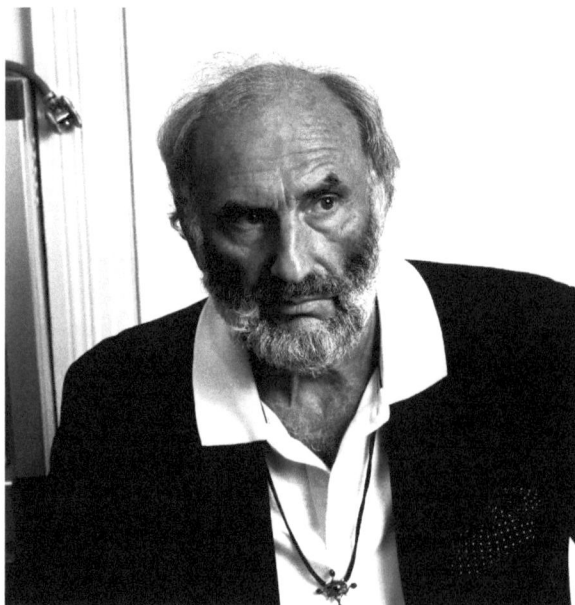

Picture 1. The Kempinski Hotel Beijing. By WhisperToMe - Own work, CC0, https://commons.wikimedia.org/w/index.php?curid=22221560

Picture 2. It shows the acupuncture treatment at the Xuan-Wu Hospital in Beijing.

Picture 3. It displays an acupuncture treatment in clinical setting.

Picture 4. It depicts the Homunculus, the map of your body "small man" or "small woman" in your brain.

Picture 5. It displays the Conception and Governing Vessels building the brain meridian and its relation to the Solar- and Pelvic plexus.

Picture 6. It displays the Conception Vessel and its relation to the Solar- and Pelvic plexus.

Picture 7. It is an Illustration of the yin-yang forces.

Picture 8. This is the image of Dr. Hua Tuo in his ancient clinical practice, painted by an unknown artist.

Picture 9. It is an illustration of an acupuncture treatment with the needles placed on Dr Hua Tuo's points alongside the spine.

Picture 10. The image displays Dr Li and Dr George, with their families in Beijing in 2013. On the right is the Sunflower, our interpreter and friend.

Picture 11. It is a modern artist's vision of the electromagnetic impact of acupuncture.

Picture 12. It illustrates the selected acupuncture points with energy channels forming a network on the leg. The hand performing the acupuncture is Dr. Li's, and the leg belongs to the author. The picture was taken in the train as we traveled to deliver the acupuncture lectures in Germany.

Picture 13. It displays the brain meridian and the flow of vital energy while you practice orbital breathing.

Picture 14. It is epicting a section through the diffusion weighted MRI of a brain. Section generated at Johns Hopkins University on 19 January 2016. Author Mim.cis. Own work. Wikipedia.

Picture 15. It illustrates how Dr. George begins the treatment with the 30 Needles Constellation Acupuncture in a clinical setting.

Picture 16. It illustrates a needle at the pivotal acupuncture point GV20 Baihui, located at the top of the head on the brain meridian.

Picture 17. It displays the Homunculus, a "neurological map" illustrating how different regions of your brain correspond to specific motor and sensory functions throughout your body.

Picture 18. This picture displays the acupuncture on the extra-point ShiShenCong with inserted needles.

Picture 19. It displays the first stage of the 30 Needles Constellation Acupuncture with all 12 needles inserted in the face and head.

Picture 20. It displays the location of the acupuncture point H7, Shenmen on the heart energy channel.

Picture 21. It displays a needle inserted in the acupuncture point H7 of the heart energy channel.

Picture 22. It displays the location of the acupuncture point L7 of the lung energy channel.

Picture 23. It displays a needle inserted at the acupuncture point L7 of the lung energy channel.

Picture 24. Lance Corporal Anthony M. Madonia emerges from the water during the swimming portion of the triathlon. Marines and Sailors of Marine Security Company and the Naval Support Facility in Thurmont, Maryland, participated in the Catoctin Mountain Triathlon

Credit: Cpl. Earnest J. Barnes, Public domain, via Wikimedia Commons.

Picture 25. Acupuncture needles are inserted at the acupuncture points LI4 Hegu of the large intestine energy channel.

Picture 26. A needle is inserted at the acupuncture point LI4 Hegu of the large intestine energy channel.

Picture 27. It displays the energy channel of the large intestine. Point LI4 is located on the hand in the valley between the thumb and index finger.

Picture 28. The large intestine energy channel course features the marked acupuncture points LI11, known as Quchi.

Picture 29. It displays a needle is inserted at point LI11, located on the large intestine energy channel.

Picture 30. It displays all 8 inserted acupuncture needled accomplishing the stage two of the 30 Needles Constellation Acupuncture.

Picture 31. It displays the stomach energy channel. Acupuncture points ST36 are marked.

Picture 32. The image depicts an inserted needle at the acupuncture point ST36 of the stomach energy channel. Additionally, the needles at the points SP6 of   the spleen energy channel above the ankle, and the K3 point of the kidney energy channel between the ankle bone and Achilles ligament are   displayed.

Picture 33. The needles 23 and 24 are inserted at the acupuncture points GB34 Yuanglinquan of the gall bladder energy channel.

Picture 34. It displays the gallbladder energy channel. The acupuncture points GB34 is marked.

Picture 35. It displays the needles inserted at the acupuncture points K3 and SP6.

Picture 36. It displays the kidney energy channel. The acupuncture points K3 are marked.

Picture 37. It displays the spleen energy channel. The acupuncture points SP6 are marked.

Picture 38. It displays acupuncture needles inserted in the points SP6.

Picture 40. The needles are inserted at points LIV3 of the liver energy channel.

Picture 41. It displays the GV26 point, "The Centre" of the brain meridian.

Picture 42. It displays the Microcosmic orbit by Bostjan46. Own work, CC0, https://commons. Wikimedia.

Picture 43. It depicts the muscle armoring.

Picture 44. It displays the acupuncture needles at the points LI20 of the large intestine energy channel, on the cheeks, beside the nose. The needles are also   inserted in the extrapoint ShiShenCong at the top of the head and in the extra-point Taiyang at the temples.

Picture 45. It displays the large intestine energy channel. The acupuncture points LI20 and LI4 are marked.